THE 30-DAY SMOOTHIE PLAN.

GET BACK ON TRACK WITHOUT PUTTING YOUR LIFE ON HOLD.

BEFORE:

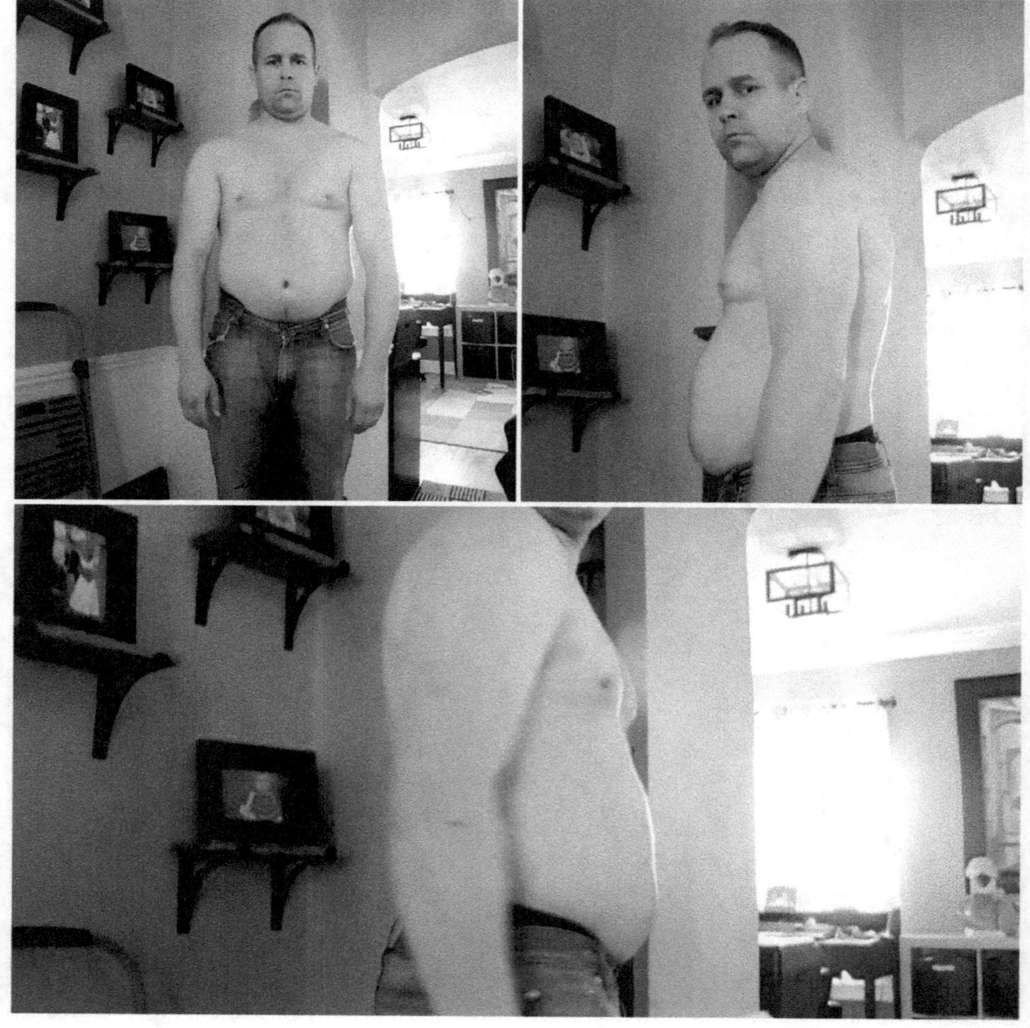

A F T E R:

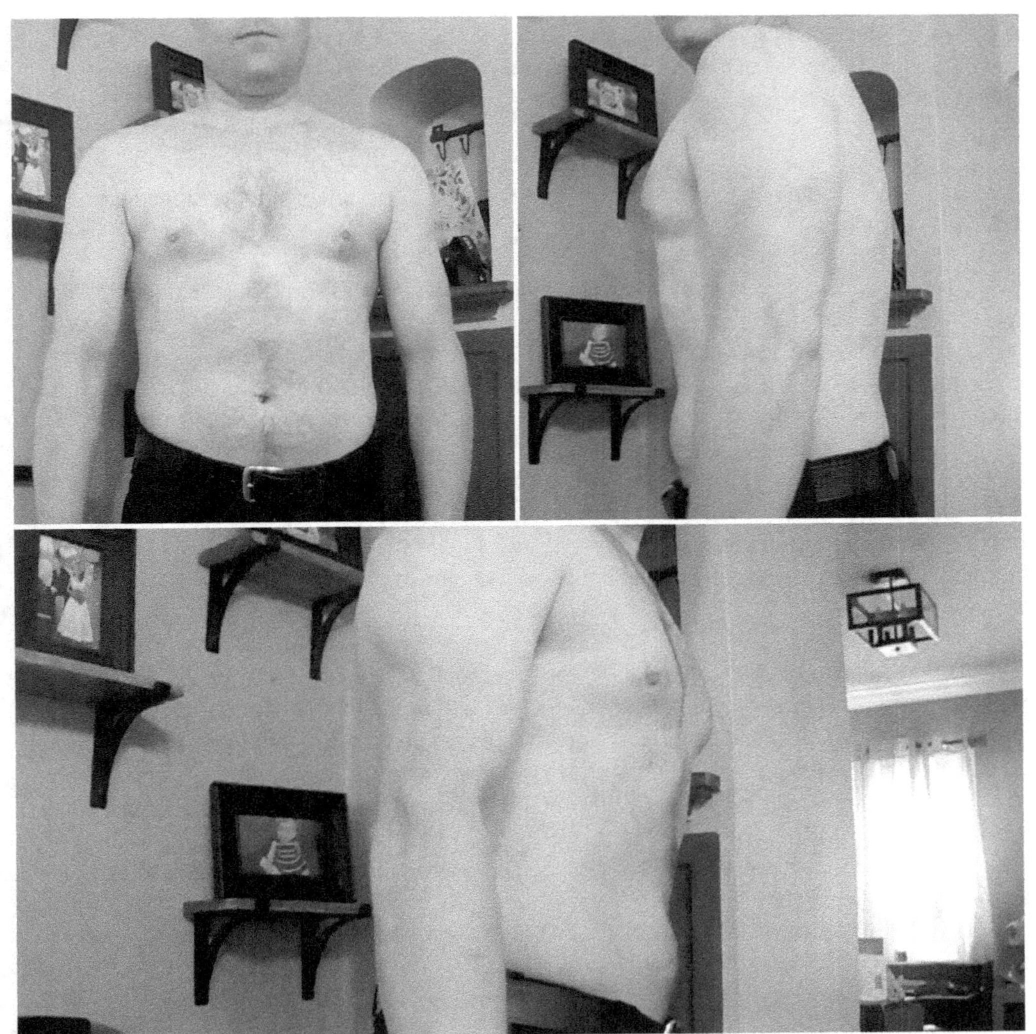

INTRODUCTION.

Welcome. I'm sure you are here because you have thought about doing a smoothie fast before, or because you have health concerns, or because you are simply looking for ways to feel better naturally. Any of these are great sources of motivation, because taking care of your body is perhaps the surest way to feeling better naturally.

In this book, I will talk about how I have made strides at achieving these same goals by doing a 30 day smoothie fast, and how it has allowed me to experience some amazing and noticeable benefits.

However, I want to start by saying that this is not a miracle-cure book. It does not offer alternatives to seeing a doctor. It does not attempt to prescribe or replace any medications, treat, heal, or cure any diseases, or solve any of the world's problems. If you have a health concern of any kind, talk to your physician. Do not delay. I am only trying to help you improve your life naturally, which is something that would benefit any living person on this planet.

So, now that that's out of the way, let's talk about why our health is important. As they say, "Health is everything. If you ain't got your health, you ain't got nothing!" Or, something like that. However the saying goes, I can honestly attest to its validity, being that I have seen firsthand the symptoms of many unhealthy people who have neglected their sleep, nutrition, and exercise needs.

In my training to be a paramedic, I was prepared to see many tragic things. You can probably imagine. However, what my training didn't prepare me for is all of the chronic illness sufferers I would witness day in and day out – people who have had amputations due to poor circulation, people who depend on machines to survive, and people who simply can no longer do what once came easy. Walking. Talking. Going to the bathroom without needing assistance.

Some of these people now have nothing but time on their hands to stare at the ceiling, contemplating life. Wondering if their illnesses were preventable and wishing they could just go back to an earlier time and take better care of themselves. Because, no amount of rebuilding can do what an ounce of prevention does.

To witness so many of these unfortunate cases has had a profound effect on me. Especially since, in the past few years, I have begun to witness the effect of my own body's neglect, telling me that I could eventually end up in the same unfortunate situation if I don't change my lifestyle soon. This has been a large part of my motivation for doing a smoothie fast, which is what we'll talk about next.

WHY I DECIDED TO DO A SMOOTHIE FAST.

Allow me to give you a brief background on myself. My name is Caleb. I am from the Chicago area, but I now live in Wisconsin. I consider myself a pretty normal guy. I have no serious illnesses, I live on a pretty average American diet, and I do an average amount of exercise.

I am 39 years old. I am 5 foot 10 inches tall. This spring, when I stepped on the scale, I weighed a total of 208 pounds. This may not seem like a lot, but for me, it is. Especially since I only weighed 40 lbs less (165 pounds) in high school when I had already finished growing.

At the start of this year (2017), my body mass index measured out at 29.8, which classified me as overweight. According to the American Heart Association, this put me at higher risk for high blood pressure, type 2 diabetes, high cholesterol, and many other serious health concerns.

I have a strong family history of coronary artery disease, rheumatoid arthritis, diabetes, and atherosclerosis on my mom's side of the family. And, on my dad's side of the family, cancer and dementia have already claimed (or impaired) a few lives. I even lost an uncle of only 53 years to a severe heart attack.

So, there are quite a few factors suggesting that I am not the type of guy (if there is such a type) who can afford to throw health-caution to the wind. I suppose it's also why, in the last few years, I have begun to grow concerned over the growing number of symptoms that I have started to notice in my body.

At some point, I had developed an irregular heartbeat. My palms and feet had become chronically sweaty. I was commonly feeling fatigued and exhausted for no apparent reason and my ability to concentrate (or remember things) was seriously lacking. I was even starting to notice psoriasis on certain parts of my skin and arthritis pain in various joints on my body.

Naturally, I did what any concerned person would do. I scheduled an appointment with my family physician, as well as a cardiologist. Unfortunately though, no diagnoses were ever made. Nor was I able to find out anything conclusive as to why I might be feeling the way I was.

So, I chalked it up to "getting older," and decided that maybe I should just learn to get used to feeling awful all the time. Somehow, it seemed like the only sensible choice I had left.

One day, I came across an amazing documentary, called "Fat, Sick, & Nearly Dead." In it, an Australian man named Joe Cross goes on a juice fast for 60 days. Afterwards, he feels (and looks) significantly better. He even claims that his regimen helped him get off of his prescription meds.

The film inspired me, and I decided to take an honest look in the mirror and acknowledge the true state of my health. It was time to quit lying to myself about what is "normal." The truth is, my problems weren't normal. I had only gotten used to living with them. And, I had become quite set in my ways.

So, I decided that, like Joe, I would embark on a journey for my own health. I decided to go on a 30-day diet of eating nothing but smoothies made of fresh fruits and vegetables. I sat down and thought about all the barriers that might get in my way, and I began to form a plan. I knew it would be hard, but I also believed that it would be worth it.

Once I was ready, I set sail on the smoothie seas. And, after 30 days, I was blown away by my results. The effects I experienced were physical, emotional, and mental. I lost over 25 lbs. My hands and feet were no longer chronically sweaty. My joints felt better too, both because they were less inflamed and because I had less body weight burdening them. I felt less stressed and anxious and as though I had been given a sense of control over my body and my life.

Now, I would love to share with you how you can experience some of the same benefits that I have! First though, let's talk about a few important things. To start, let's ask the question:

WHY 30 DAYS?

This is a good question. There are many different smoothie books and plans out there. Some of them are only three, five, nine, or ten days in duration. Why did I pick the number thirty? At first, simply because it seemed like a fair and rounded number.

Joe did a sixty day juice fast, but, unlike him, I do not have the luxury of taking large amounts of time away from my job to focus purely on my health. Someday, I might, but for now, I have to keep balancing life while trying to make changes in my lifestyle.

Because of this, I figured that the number thirty was a more realistic number to aim for. It is a small enough amount of time to reasonably commit to, and yet, a long enough amount of time to achieve the desired effects on the body.

WHY SMOOTHIES? ISN'T JUICING BETTER?

Juices and smoothies are similar, but they differ in a few ways. One of the main concepts behind juicing is that you give your GI tract a break, which provides your body with a lot of extra energy that it would normally delegate to the rigorous task of digestion. When you do a smoothie fast, you do not get this benefit. At least, not to the same degree.

However, you do get all of the benefits of eating tons of fiber and vitamin-filled ingredients which can help your body in the exact same way. And, they are blended, which means that your body doesn't have to work nearly as hard to digest them.

Plus, most people find juicing to be a much bigger hassle. Not only is a juicer harder to clean, it utilizes only a small portion of the produce you put in it. A blender utilizes everything you put into it. Nothing goes to waste!

WHAT DOES THE 30 DAY SMOOTHIE PLAN CONSIST OF?

The main aspects of the 30 day smoothie plan are as follows:

A. Smoothies only for 30 days.
B. 8 hours of sleep every night.
C. Light exercise every day.
D. Less media than you normally consume.
E. Less caffeine than you normally consume.
F. No alcohol.
G. Large amounts of purified water.
H. Elimination of sugar, salt, soy, dairy, corn, gluten, meat, eggs.
I. Elimination of MSG, GMOs, artificial flavors, high-fructose sweeteners, and partially hydrogenated oils.
J. 1 trip to the supermarket every week.

As you can see, the plan is pretty simple. But, simple and easy are two very different things. Don't be fooled into thinking that this won't require a complete lifestyle change. At least, temporarily.

Smoothies are the main part of the plan, and the word "Smoothie" alone may conjure up a plethora of different images. It may make you think of a gooey green slime concocted by Bill Nye the Science Guy. Or, a blend of Oreos and ice cream served up by your local ice cream guy. To be clear about what a smoothie is (or at least, which kind we will be drinking), I could best sum it up by saying that it should include all natural, fresh, and healthy ingredients.

It should not have any added dairy, salt, or sugar. Maybe this goes without saying, but then again, maybe it doesn't. No dairy because of the way it is produced and because it is something that many people are sensitive to – a lot of them, unknowingly.

While it is impossible to completely avoid salt and sugar, being that they are naturally found in the fruits and vegetables we will be blending, our smoothies will not contain any added sugar or salt. Even the juices we will use as a base will contain more sugar than is ideal.

So, when you are at the store, picking out your juices and any other ingredients, please keep this in mind. Try to avoid things that have any added sugar. You should DEFINITELY avoid it if it contains any high-fructose sweeteners.

I should give the disclaimer that the recipes in this book include apple juice and freshly squeezed orange juice. They also use more fruits than vegetables. If you'd like, you can substitute these ingredients for others that you feel would work better for you. Feel free to get creative with your variety. Just make sure that whatever you choose is healthy!

As for the total amount of smoothie that you should blend each day, I have found that, for myself, sixty four ounces of smoothie will suffice perfectly. This plan works under the assumption that most people are like me, and will consume roughly the same amount. Of course, you may require more (or fewer) calories than me. If that is the case, I recommend that you modify your plan accordingly.

This plan uses recipes that will each make about sixty four ounces of smoothie! If you ration them out at a reasonable pace throughout each day (alternating between smoothie and water consumption), my recipes ought to work well for you!

As you went through all that this plan involves, you probably noticed that it involved much more than just smoothies. For one, I included sleep as an aspect we would focus on. I chose to include this because, much like the way we neglect nutrition, we neglect how important it is for our bodies to get adequate rest.

I recently discovered that sleep debt is defined as "Going more than two days in a row with less than seven hours of sleep." Ouch. According to this, I have been in sleep debt my whole life. So has nearly every person I've ever known! Wouldn't it be nice to experience what it's like not to be in sleep debt for a while?

You may choose to make sleep a priority as well, and I advise that you do. Not only is it physically beneficial, it can do even more. Because, since most of our intense food urges come at night, we can go to bed early and sleep right through those times when we'd otherwise be tempted to break all of our rules in indulgent streaks of binging.

Also, you'll see that the plan includes light exercise each day. This is because the average person neglects exercise too. As for myself, I can say this is true. I have a somewhat sedentary lifestyle and spend way too much time sitting around at work.

By light exercise, I don't mean spending four hours at the gym every day. The caloric intake of this diet alone make that idea unreasonable. Rather, I'm suggesting that it would be good to get up off the couch and go for a walk or a short run each day. Do something that makes you break a sweat. Don't overdo it, but don't underdo it either.

The plan also involves consuming less media. I included this because, well, it's just not good for us to be on our phones and computers so much. Think about all the time we spend with our eyes glued to tiny, bright screens, stuck in an almost trancelike state.

This is time that could be spent growing or reflecting on life's important matters. And, since we're already training ourselves to take a break from most all other guilty pleasures, why not take a break from this too?

And now, caffeine. Yup, I said it. I know this may seem like an impossible thing to give up. And to be honest, not even I was willing to give it up during my thirty days (even though I believe it would have been the wisest option). Maybe you'll do better.

Or, maybe you're just as hard-headed as me, in which case, you may choose to at least cut way back on the amount that you consume. Again, I don't know what the experts would say about this. Some might find it preposterous that I would even have a sip of coffee during a smoothie fast. I'm not saying you should. I'm just saying that I did and I still managed to achieve all of my fitness and weight-loss goals. If you aren't sure what to do, run it by your physician.

Also, stay away from all alcohol during this thirty day period. While it is arguable that there are certain health benefits to a glass of red wine, your body will already have enough to endure with all of these strange changes. Not to mention, your stomach will be less full than it usually is and any alcohol will have a much stronger effect. So, please stay away from it.

Of course, as always, drink plenty of water. I find that, on a normal day, I don't usually drink enough of it. Even my coworkers have noticed this and mentioned it to me. So, I have recognized the need to pay attention to how much water I'm getting and to be sure I get enough. Especially during this period!

Many of us binge drink water, which actually isn't very helpful. When we wake up, we slam an entire liter, thinking that we've met our days requirements in one fell swoop. Wrong. The truth is that we need to be sipping water regularly throughout the day. If you'd like to do as I have done, simply keep a gallon of purified water close by. That way, you have enough to last you.

To make this plan run smoothly, you'll need to make one trip to the supermarket each week. I'm assuming that you have a refrigerator, right? Good! Later on, I will provide you with a list of all that you'll need to fill it with. If you get all of the ingredients that are on that list, you should not have to worry about running low on supply each week.

As you can see, the plan involves quite a few variables. And, should you choose to follow it to its entirety, I believe you'll find that the combination of all these variables work with each other almost synergistically to bring restoration to your body from all angles.

You may only choose to commit to the smoothie aspect of the plan. Or, you may choose to follow the plan entirely. However you choose to go about it is up to you. But, for the best possible outcome, I recommend going for the gold. In other words, following it to the tee.

Before starting, you should take into consideration any of your own special needs. If you have diabetes, a heart condition, or any other health concern that could be adversely affected, talk about it with your doctor before starting this (or any other) health plan.

Even if you don't have a preexisting condition that you are aware of, talk to your physician anyway. Be sure to share all that it involves and follow any advice you are given. You can't be too careful with your body. After all, good self-care and wholeness are the whole goal of this book. My aim is to help you reach that goal, not compromise it.

WHAT YOU'LL NEED:

A. A good blender. (I recommend either a Vitamix, Nutribullet, or Blendtec, even though there are many other great blenders out there that are available for a reasonable price).
B. Fresh juices (or bases) and produce that you've picked up ahead of time (In the weekly lists provided).
C. A journal (provided in the paperback version of this book).
D. Thermoses or coolers that you can use to contain your smoothies and keep them cool throughout the day.
E. A plan that works specifically with your life.

THE RECIPES:

Here are the five smoothie recipes that you can use throughout the month, should you care to use them. Each smoothie makes roughly 64 fluid ounces (or half of a gallon) and can be made solely by using the ingredients on the list which you've picked up from the store at the beginning of each week.

Of course, you can use your own recipes if you'd like. I only provide these recipes as a way to make your life simpler. If you use them, you can also use the chart I have provided below. It'll keep your smoothies alternating in such a way that you never repeat them consecutively.

You may decide that you like one of these smoothie ideas but not the others. You may decide that you like all but one, or none of them at all. You may even decide to give them your own unique touch. If you see something you like, which in your opinion, could use a dash of something else, go for it. Just remember to revise your grocery list accordingly, because the list I provide will only work with the five smoothie recipes I have included.

Lastly, please take into account that you will have to add to your list any additional flavorings, supplements, probiotic powders, or vitamin mixes that you choose to use. The types, contents, and flavors to choose from are many. Look for good quality and good flavor, because you want something that you will enjoy. And, make sure you buy enough of it to last you.

SMOOTHIE CHART

Day 1 Smoothie recipe #1	Day 2 Smoothie recipe #2	Day 3 Smoothie recipe #3	Day 4 Smoothie recipe # 4	Day 5 Smoothie recipe #5
Day 6 Smoothie recipe #1	Day 7 Smoothie recipe #2	Day 8 Smoothie recipe #3	Day 9 Smoothie recipe # 4	Day 10 Smoothie recipe #5
Day 11 Smoothie recipe #1	Day 12 Smoothie recipe #2	Day 13 Smoothie recipe #3	Day 14 Smoothie recipe # 4	Day 15 Smoothie recipe #5
Day 16 Smoothie recipe #1	Day 17 Smoothie recipe #2	Day 18 Smoothie recipe #3	Day 19 Smoothie recipe # 4	Day 20 Smoothie recipe #5
Day 21 Smoothie recipe #1	Day 22 Smoothie recipe #2	Day 23 Smoothie recipe #3	Day 24 Smoothie recipe # 4	Day 25 Smoothie recipe #5
Day 26 Smoothie recipe #1	Day 27 Smoothie recipe #2	Day 28 Smoothie recipe #3	Day 29 Smoothie recipe # 4	Day 30 Smoothie recipe #5

5 SMOOTHIE RECIPES

Smoothie Recipe #1.   THE GARDENER
(Days 1,6,11,16,21,26)

1 avocado = 3oz
1 cup spinach = 2oz
1 cup kale = 3oz
1 apple = 5oz
1 kiwi = 3oz
1 carrot = 3oz
1 cup of strawberries = 7oz
1 cup of raspberries = 8oz
3 cups apple juice = 24oz

Smoothie Recipe #2.   THE QUAKER
(Days 2,7,12,17,22,27)

1 avocado = 3 oz
1 cup of oatmeal (Gluten free) = 3 oz
3 apples = 15 oz
½ cup raisins = 3 oz
A dash of cinnamon
1 cup of raw almonds = 8 oz
2 cups of spinach 4 oz
3 cups of almond milk 24 oz

Smoothie Recipe #3.   THE CHOCOLATE DAYDREAM
(Days 3,8,13,18,23,28)

1 kiwi = 3 oz
1 cup of blueberries = 8 oz
1 Banana = 4 oz
2 cup spinach = 4 oz
3 oranges = 15 oz
2 cup almond milk = 16 oz
1 cup orange juice = 8 oz
2 scoops chocolate vegan protein mix for flavoring.

Smoothie Recipe #4.   THE PROBIOTIC BLAST
(Days 4,9,14,19,24,29)

1 kiwi = 3 oz
1 banana = 4 oz
2 oranges = 10 oz
1 cup spinach = 2 oz

1 cup of raspberries = 8 oz
1 cup of blueberries = 8 oz
1 cup almond milk = 8 oz
2 cups orange juice = 16 oz
1 scoop probiotic powder

Smoothie Recipe #5.   THE ISLANDER
(Days 5,10,15,20,25,30)

1 kiwi = 3 oz
2 oranges = 10 oz
1 banana = 4 oz
2 mango = 12 oz
1 cup diced pineapple = 6 oz
1 cup kale = 3 oz
2 cups of coconut milk = 16 oz
1 cup orange juice = 8 oz
(Optional - add 1 scoop of chocolate vegan protein mix).

CAN I REALLY GET ALL THE NUTRIENTS I NEED FROM FRUIT AND VEGETABLES?

This is another great question. The smoothie plan that I have presented is purely vegan. Actually, it is an elimination diet of sorts, because it does more than simply eliminate meat. It also eliminates many of the other foods that people are sensitive to, such as salt, soy, dairy, corn, gluten, eggs, and excess sugar.

By eliminating these foods, we are further eliminating most of the byproducts that are found in processed foods, such as MSG, hormones, some GMOs, high-fructose sweeteners, and partially hydrogenated oils. If you choose to go organic, you'll do even better at this elimination!

Of course, you may be concerned about how this diet also eliminates certain good things, such as calcium, protein, and iron, which we normally rely on meat and dairy for. Fear not. If you would like to maintain your normal intake of these things, you can find vegan supplements which include them at your local health food store. Many of these supplements will not only enhance the content to your smoothies, but the flavor as well!

While there is a lot of science on both sides of the vegan argument, many studies have been done which suggest that the vegan lifestyle can be both beneficial and healing. Some of my favorite supportive studies include: *The China Study, The Gerson Therapy*, and of course, the documentary I mentioned, called *Fat, Sick, & Nearly Dead.*

On a personal level, I have talked to many people who have gone vegan and experienced some amazing effects from it. They include my mom, my brother, and a few close friends, who all have experienced some very positive results from going vegan, such as looking better, feeling better, and having more energy.

ENSURING YOUR SUCCESS -

PREPARING FOR CHALLENGES -

As you've probably already begun to notice, this journey is challenging. Obviously, it will challenge you physically. But, it will challenge you in even more ways – emotionally, mentally, financially, socially, logistically, and even spiritually.

On the physical side of things, your body has probably built up a tolerance (as well as an addiction) to all sorts of synthetic nonsense. When you cut yourself off from these things, you may experience a type of withdrawal, which, as we know, can be a painful, difficult process. It may come with headaches, nausea, fatigue, and irritability.

It may feel like your body is protesting, and actually, it will be. It probably has forgotten what it was meant to run on (ie, real food), and it has probably forgotten the way it was meant to feel (ie, not constantly fatigued and sore). So, it's kind of like they say… it gets worse before it gets better.

On the emotional side of things, you may begin to experience some anxiety or depression. After all, you are taking something away from your diet that once gave you an unnatural immediate rush of joy or comfort. Now, without that, you can expect to feel some of the bad emotions that you were burying beneath fast food Band-Aids.

Not to get all mushy-gushy here, but there is a spiritual side to this as well. Because, when you do this, you are doing something that is hard, which requires discipline and self-denial. You are learning to tune out urges that you have normally succumbed to.

I can't help but think of the Bible verse that says: "He who can conquer his spirit is mightier than he who can conquer a city." In other words, the real mountaintops we seek to ascend aren't out there in the Himalayas… they are within us, involving our fears, temptations, and doubts.

Whether or not you believe in the Bible, you can probably at least agree that there is virtue in abstaining from certain pleasures, and a lot of good that can come from it. Good things are never easy, and being intentional about developing your own willpower will help you in EVERY area of life – at work, in parenting, and in all of your relationships.

Regarding the social aspect of this plan, there is more to consider. Because, once you start to change your lifestyle, people around you will start to notice. Some will start giving you lectures about what you are doing. Others will suddenly start acting like experts on the subjects of nutrition, health, and moderation.

I advise you not to be offended and to take what they say with a grain of salt. Most of them are only speaking out of genuine concern. However, there are those who will take your actions personally. They'll think you are arrogant for choosing not to sit down and join them at the dinner table. Again, take it with a grain of salt.

Thirty days later, these will be the same people asking you what your secret is and how you managed to look and feel so much better in such a short amount of time. It's amazing how minds tend to open up after witnessing great transformations.

If you feel that there are certain people in your life that will not be understanding or encouraging to you on this journey, you may want to figure out a way to distance yourself from them during this period.

We should mention that there is a mental aspect to this journey as well, as it will challenge you to think differently than you have in the past. You'll have to form new perspectives and refrain from slipping back into "autopilot."   And, you'll find that you can gain a lot of mental strength by learning to take control over circumstances that you once thought you were helpless in.

On the financial side of things, consider all of the costs involved. Unless you have a natural garden of lush fruits and vegetables that is accessible to you year round, you will have to pay for good produce, and the costs can add up.

Logistically, this will affect you as well. Especially if you're anything like me, having a marriage, a mortgage, a family, and a full-time job to sustain, you'll find that it isn't always easy to juggle another ball. This journey does indeed require some daily planning, which is why we so easily find ourselves in the drive-thru lane. Forming a new lifestyle will require you to figure out how to make it all work. Fortunately, I have done a lot of that work for you in this book!

MAKING YOURSELF ACCOUNTABLE.

Can you do this on your own? Probably, but why? Wouldn't it be better to have people nearby who can encourage you and help keep you accountable? I recommend that you tell a few trusted friends or family members what you are up to and have them check in with you periodically. If you want, you can even make videos on a regular basis to update people on your progress.

To ensure my chances of success, I did just that. When I mentioned on my Facebook page that I would be doing the fast, I also said that I would be posting videos of my progress as I went along. This turned out to be a great decision.

Because, when you know you have to face the world about your actions, you become a little bit more motivated to keep your promises, as well as to keep your mistakes to a bare minimum.

We all get motivated, and then we all seem to watch our motivation melt like a popsicle in the desert. So, the decision to stay accountable worked wonders for me, because at times, it was my only motivation to keep going.

The most important thing to realize is that your inspiration will waver, especially with all of the unseen challenges that you'll face. Temptation is like a bandit, waiting to ambush you at every turn. If you want to make it, it will be of enormous help to have any added incentives you can find.

If you care to watch any of the videos I have made, I will post links to them in my daily journal which you will be able to access near your own journal entries, should you decide to make any. I recommend that you do, because this will be a period of growth for you. You will want to remember what you learned in it.

COMING UP WITH YOUR OWN MOTIVATIONAL LIST OF REASONS.

Because of all of the challenges we've talked about, I recommend that you make a list of all of your reasons for doing a smoothie fast. You should include your health goals, as well as any health concerns that you would like to see improved.

Read and reread your list every day. It will be an important source of motivation for you as you go along. Especially when that triple cheeseburger is staring you in the face and you can't remember why you have decided to say no to it.

KEEPING A JOURNAL.

Journaling is a good stress reliever. A lot of times, when we take the time to put our thoughts and feelings into words, it clarifies things for us and has an almost therapeutic effect. That is why I have included journaling as a primary part of this journey. I highly recommend that you set aside a few times each day to write in your journal.

Alongside your own journal entries, I have included my own. This way, you can look over at mine as you go along. It will help to see my thoughts next to yours so that you feel a sense of rhythm. It may even relieve you to see that my emotional roller coaster is similar to yours. Hopefully, it gives you the sense that you are not alone in this.

I also will include motivational thoughts for each day. Some of them are the thoughts of other people that I have found encouraging. Others, I have come up with on my own. All of these thoughts and ideas are there to help inspire you along the way, just as they have done for me.

If you have purchased the paperback version of this book, then the journal will be easy to use. Just open up to whichever day you are on and start scribbling away. However, if you have the Kindle version of this book, it will be difficult to use the journal, as Kindle books aren't designed to be written in.

If that's the case for you, I recommend that you make a Word doc with the questions below and print out 30 copies. Then, you will have every day covered. Be sure to give yourself adequate amounts of spacing between the questions so that you are able to pencil in your entries without problem.

Check in 1: 10am (or after)

- What are my main concerns and predictions for the day?
- Also, were yesterday's concerns/predictions accurate?
- How many hours of sleep did I get?
- Did I drink enough water yesterday?
- What am I learning and experiencing?
- How can I apply what I am learning?

Check in 2: 6pm (or after)

- Have I succeeded in my daily goals so far?

- How I feel so far (Emotionally, physically, relationally, etc):
- Problems I am encountering and how I am dealing with them:
- What was the most difficult part of the day?
- What should I learn to do differently tomorrow (and in the future) to help me stay on track?
- What have I found helpful?

OTHER DAILY QUESTIONS YOU MAY WANT TO INCLUDE -

What was my weight at the start of the day? __________
Do you notice any abnormalities/differences? _____________________
What did you put in your smoothie?___________
Have you done any light exercise? Yes or no.
Have you absorbed less media? Yes or no.
Did you have regular bowel movements?
Have you immersed yourself in any pertinent inspirational material? Yes or no.
Do you feel that you planned/prepared adequately for the day?___________
What might you have done differently? ________________

WEANING YOURSELF OFF OF (AND BACK ONTO) FOOD.

As we move closer towards actually starting, we should talk about one more important thing. It happens to be another thing I didn't do (that you should), which is: make the transition into fasting gently. The night before my fast began, I filled my stomach to the rafters with Easter food. Apparently, this is a big no-no, and it wasn't long before I got to see why.

My first day was miserable, as you'll find out later in my journal (if you care to read it). I had a stomach ache. I had a headache and felt nauseous and irritable. Of course, this is for a number of different reasons.

For one, my body wasn't yet used to all the nutrients of a strictly plant-based diet. Also, it was used to being packed with excessive amounts of sugar, salt, and processed foods. Moreover, my stomach walls went from being stretched to their max to being nearly empty in a short period of time, which can be extremely painful. In hindsight, I would have done this much differently.

As Joe recommends, you should start getting your body accustomed one week before starting, changing the way you eat so that your body starts getting ready.

During this week, he advises you to cut out junk food, processed meats, dairy, and soda, and to make your portion sizes smaller. Also, to start adding foods that are good for you and easy to digest, such as salads, soups, whole foods, fruits, nuts, and vegetables. Also, be sure to start drinking plenty of water.

Remember that all of these same principles will apply once you are done with your fast and ready to reenter the world of solid foods. In other words, don't go to the all-you-can-eat buffet to celebrate on your first night back. Or, during that whole first week, for that matter.

In fact, stick to a plant-based diet during that first week back. Eat some of the produce that you're used to throwing in a blender. An apple. A banana. Or, have a soup or a fresh salad, but remember to watch your portion sizes.

Remember to chew your food really well too. The work you do in your mouth decreases the work your stomach has to do in digesting. Drink lots of water and stay away from alcohol. You'll find that you don't need much sugar or salt in order to make your food taste great.

Stay moving. If you've done your share of light exercise throughout the month, keep at it. Don't stop doing what has been working so well to make you feel better, sharper, and lighter.

Take your time going back to food. You may even want to figure out which foods not to go back to at all.

This is a great opportunity to make some positive life changes that will stick! After all, you are already used to a stricter diet. Even if you were to have two smoothies a day and one sensible meal for dinner, it would be easy compared to what you've been through.

I advise anyone who does this plan to think about how they can make some positive permanent changes. Because, the truth is that most temporary health plans are just that – temporary. As soon as they end, so do the benefits. But, do you really want to regain all the weight you've lost? Do you really want to go back to feeling sluggish and drained all the time? I don't think you do, or you would never have started this plan in the first place!

FORMING A PLAN AND SCHEDULE THAT WORK FOR YOU.

So, we have discussed the benefits of this plan, our reasons for doing it, and we have a pretty good idea about what it is. If you've decided that you're on board, you just have one more major thing to figure out – **when** you would like to start. Have you given this some thought?

Now is usually the best answer when it comes to making great life changes, but in this case, there are a few things you should consider before you actually commit to starting, which will play a large part in the success of your journey.

Take a look at the calendar. Do you see any big holidays coming up? If so, you may want to avoid that time. Holidays often revolve around food and how much of it we can fill our faces with. Not that we shouldn't practice discretion during those times (or all times, for that matter), but we should be realistic about the temptations we'll face and how likely they are to throw us off track.

For the best results, look for a time frame that doesn't coincide with a barbecue at Aunt Judy's, where you'll probably be tempted to defend your title in the annual pie eating competition. If you can find a better thirty day chunk of time, choose that instead. You'll thank yourself later.

Should you decide to pick a period of time that happens to be full of big holidays and eat outs, just keep that list you've made handy. It'll be your life raft, keeping you afloat in the seas of scrumptious, edible temptations.

If, in a moment of weakness, you happen to say "Yes" when Aunt Judy offers you a piece of homemade French silk pie, don't worry. It doesn't mean you are disqualified. If you fall off the wagon, get back on it. Don't delay, or see it as an excuse to have four more pieces. One of the main enemies you'll face on this journey is discouragement.

One way to keep yourself from becoming discouraged is by thinking about what you would like to turn to *instead* of those pleasures and comforts that you'll be giving up. For example, if you plan on giving up coffee, figure out beforehand what you'll replace it with.

If you've decided that decaffeinated green tea will suffice as a replacement, make sure that you add it to your grocery list so that you have plenty of it whenever the desire (or need) for coffee might arise.

If you plan on giving up television, maybe you could replace it with exercise. If you plan on giving up phone games, maybe you could replace them with a good, motivational book to read. You could also substitute unwanted activities for time spent journaling.

I also recommend that you set reminders to keep yourself on track throughout each day. Do you have a timer on your watch or an app on your phone? These things can keep you aware of when it's time to drink more water, return to the supermarket, write in your journal, blend your smoothies, and head off to bed.

If you know you're not a morning person, then blend your smoothies the night before. Set a timer to go off at 9pm, sometime before you start getting tired. If you know that weekends are crazy, set an alarm on Friday to start preparing for the craziness ahead of time.

If you know that you aren't good at drinking water, set an alarm to go off every hour or so, reminding you to take a few sips. These small reminders will help keep you in line with your goals and give you less to think about while you focus on life's demands.

Now, before we go any further, please take a look at your calendar if you have not done so already. Set this book down. Do you see a good chunk of time that could work for you – one that not only looks good on the calendar, but that you feel emotionally ready to charge into?

If so, great! Once you get close to that day, you are ready to take:

A TRIP TO THE STORE.

So, you've been weaning yourself off of solid foods. You plan on starting sometime within the next two days. You have your phone reminders all set up. You have your recipes, a list of personal inspirations, and a pen, ready for journaling. Now, all you need is the produce! Grab your first week's grocery list and head off to the store!

I should mention that the first week's list is the most expensive, being that this is when you will be buying some of the pricier items that will last you all month, such as your probiotic and protein mixes, as well as a few other items that you will only need to purchase once. Outside of these expenses, the plan stays reasonably priced, especially when you consider that it is replacing your normal food costs.

For those of you who plan on using the chart and recipes I have provided, you will need to buy everything on the list below for week 1. If you have formed your own plan and list, and you're ready to begin, then off to the supermarket we go!

GROCERY LISTS -

WEEK 1 -

THINGS YOU MUST ONLY BUY ONCE (WHICH SHOULD LAST YOU ALL MONTH):
1 - Container of probiotic powder, flavored to your liking.
1 - Container of vegan chocolate protein mix.
1 - Large package of Quaker Gluten Free Oatmeal.
1 - Container of cinnamon (If you don't already have some).
1 - Bag of carrots (1 pound)
Any other healthy additives you would like to use

1 - 64 oz container of quality apple juice.
1 - 64 oz container of freshly squeezed orange juice.
1 - 20 oz container of raisins (preferably organic).
1 - 64 oz container of coconut milk.
2 - 64 oz containers of almond milk.
1 - Pound of raw almonds (Preferably organic).
1 - Pound of strawberries (Preferably organic).
1 - Pound of blueberries (Preferably organic).
2 - Pounds of Raspberries (Preferably organic).
3 - 6 oz bags of baby spinach (I get these from Trader Joe's).
1 - 10 oz bag of kale (This also can be found at Trader Joe's).
7 - Full sized oranges.
4 - Large avocados.
5 - Kiwis
8 - Good sized apples.

At the end of this week, you should still have:
16 oz of apple juice leftover for next week.
32 oz of orange juice leftover for next week.
14 oz of raisins leftover for next week.
44 oz of coconut milk leftover for next week.
56 oz of almond milk leftover for next week.
8 oz of raspberries leftover for next week.

WEEK 2 -

1 - 64 oz container of apple juice.
1 - Pound of raw almonds
1 - Pound of strawberries
2 - Pounds of blueberries
1 - Pound of Raspberries
3 - 6 oz bags of baby spinach
1 - 10 oz bag of kale
12 - Full sized oranges.
2 - Large avocados.
6 - Kiwis
4 - Good sized apples.
3 - Bananas

At the end of this week, you should still have:
24 oz Almond milk leftover for next week
4 oz Orange juice leftover for next week
11 oz Raisins leftover for next week
56 oz Apple Juice leftover for next week
28 oz Coconut Milk leftover for next week
8 oz Raw almonds leftover for next week
9 oz Strawberries leftover for next week
4 oz Kale leftover for next week

WEEK 3 -

1 - 64 oz Container of freshly squeezed orange juice.
1 - 64 oz Container of coconut milk.
1 - 64 oz Container of almond milk.
1 - Pound of strawberries
1 - Pound of blueberries
2 - Pounds of Raspberries
3 - 6 oz bags of baby spinach
1 - 10 oz bag of kale
9 - Full sized oranges.
3 - Large avocados.
6 - Kiwis
5 - Good sized apples.
4 - Bananas

At the end of this week, you should still have:
8 oz Apple juice leftover for next week
28 oz Orange juice leftover for next week
8 oz Raisins leftover for next week
8 oz Raspberries leftover for next week
60 oz Coconut milk leftover for next week
16 oz Almond milk leftover for next week
11 oz Strawberries leftover for next week
4 oz Spinach leftover for next week
2 oz Kale leftover for next week

WEEK 4 - (Includes shopping list for the 2 remaining days after week 4 as well)

1 - 16 oz container of apple juice.
1 - 64 oz container of freshly squeezed orange juice
2 - 64 oz containers of almond milk.
1 - Pound of raw almonds
2 - Pounds of blueberries
1 - Pound of Raspberries
2 - 6 oz bags of baby spinach
1 - 10 oz bag of kale
14 - Full sized oranges.
3 - Large avocados.
7 - Kiwis
7 - Good sized apples.
5 - Bananas

JOURNAL, DAY 1

Check in 1 (10am or later)
How many hours of sleep did I get last night? _______________
Did I drink enough water yesterday? _____________________
What am I learning and experiencing?

What are my main concerns and predictions for the day?

Were yesterday's concerns/predictions accurate?

How can I apply what I am learning?

Check in 2 (6pm or later)
Have I succeeded in my daily goals so far?

How I feel so far (Emotionally, physically, relationally, etc):

Problems I have encountered and how I am dealing with them:

What was the most difficult part (or time) of the day?

What can I learn to do differently tomorrow (and in the future) to help me stay on track?

CALEB'S JOURNAL, DAY 1 -

Check In 1 - <u>VIDEO</u>

So ,this is day one of my journey and it is 11:30 a.m. it's April 17th 2017, and it is a Monday. It happens to be the first day after Easter, which is of some significance, because Easter is about resurrection, and hopefully I will be resurrected as well in many ways.

But this also means that my stomach is full of food from eating way too much last night, and I'll probably be paying for it as the size of my stomach retracts. Going from feast to famine in one day is a change that's drastic and sudden. Hopefully, it goes well. So far, it hasn't been terrible.

Today I am at work, which will be a common thing for me on this journey, as I will be living life like I always do (with the exception of some small lifestyle changes). I'm kind of glad for this though, because I want to learn how to make these changes stick in everyday life.

Our ambulance is parked in a parking lot in Highland Park Illinois and we are experiencing some down time. Normally, I would be chowing down on a plate of biscuits and gravy, followed by a nap. Notice how none of it involves exercise, or anything healthy for that matter.

I did not make any smoothies today or bring anything with me, so I will have to go to Jamba Juice, which is a chain we have in this area and you may have to, which prepares juices and smoothies for you if you are on the go. It can be a little pricey, but it is very convenient on days like this when I failed to make adequate preparations ahead of time.

So far, my motivation has not suffered, though that may only be because this is the first day and this whole journey still feels new and exciting. I wonder if I'll still feel that way later on when I'm hungry and every Taco Bell I drive past looks like an old friend calling me over, saying "Come to me. I'm familiar. I give you comfort. I'll make you feel better." I'll have to say "No, sorry." While that moment has not yet come, I know better than to think it won't.

Check in 2: <u>VIDEO</u>

I'm not going to lie. This day has become extremely challenging. If you watch the video, you'll see what I mean. I explained it a little bit. Long story short though, when 3 o'clock p.m. rolled around, it felt like I was blindsided by a wave of strong emotions.

I suddenly became cranky and irritable. I became fidgety and restless. All I could think about was food and choosing to start my smoothie cleanse tomorrow instead of today. However, that's the kind of thinking I've had for many years now, and I am determined not to give in.

Today, while I was experiencing this wide array of emotions, I walked into a hospital and noticed in the nurses lounge that there was a smorgasbord of free food sitting on a credenza in the break station. It took every bit of willpower I had not to charge in there and fill up my gut. Of course, free food only seems to find me when I'm dieting. Anyway.

It all gave me an interesting thought. It made me realize that food is a comfort, but anytime we want comfort, there's something we want to be comforted from. When you choose to take an aspirin it is because you have a headache. But, here's the interesting thing - it doesn't really make the headache go away. It just covers it up for a while. Maybe the food we turn to for comfort is the same. And maybe, once the effect of our comfort food wears off, the initial pain and anxiety that we tried to bury begins to resurface. Maybe this is a good chance to discover things in me that need to be dealt with. Just a thought.

JOURNAL, DAY 2

Check in 1 (10am or later)
How many hours of sleep did I get last night? _______________
Did I drink enough water yesterday? _________________________
What am I learning and experiencing?

What are my main concerns and predictions for the day?

Were yesterday's concerns/predictions accurate?

How can I apply what I am learning?

Check in 2 (6pm or later)
Have I succeeded in my daily goals so far?

How I feel so far (Emotionally, physically, relationally, etc):

Problems I have encountered and how I am dealing with them:

What was the most difficult part (or time) of the day?

What can I learn to do differently tomorrow (and in the future) to help me stay on track?

CALEB'S JOURNAL, DAY 2 -

If you become uninspired, remember that your list of reasons is your inspiration. Every single thing on that list is a reminder of why you are doing this and points to a potential area for improvement in your life. Look at your list as often as you need to.

Check in 1: <u>VIDEO</u>

I think I mentioned yesterday that it's funny how free food seems to pop up whenever you go on a diet. It's as though the universe knows you are trying to stay away from something and decides to make it free when you don't want it.

My wife even bought me a rice crispy treat out of the blue and set it on the counter for me with a note that says "Just because." While it is a very sweet notion, it too seems ironically timed. Thanks universe, but I know what you're up to.

This morning has been challenging, but not so much in a food-sense. It's been challenging in a busyness-sense – trying to manage my day-to-day responsibilities. Three days a weak I'm a stay-at-home dad with both of my daughters, which can be a full-time job.

Even though no food cravings have come yet, I don't want to be naive, because I know that most of them come at night. So, if I can stay on track until then, I will hopefully have enough momentum going to make it through the night.

To enhance my smoothie even more, I've added a chocolate vegan protein mix, and it is delicious! It's amazing what a little chocolate will do to correct an off-balance mix. I think I may be onto something long-term here.

I didn't get a full 8 hours of sleep last night. Probably more like 6 and a half, and it was frequently interrupted. I ended up coming home late from work and there's nothing I can do when that happens. I'm simply stuck with whatever I can get.

On another note, I noticed that some of my arthritis pain was gone this morning. I think that even a small break from normal food can make big differences in matters of inflammation.

Today ought to go a little smoother than yesterday. At least, I hope. This time I will not be relying on smoothie stores. I have my own supply and enough of it to last me. I also have a gallon of water which I will be drinking throughout the day.

Check in 2: <u>VIDEO</u>

I had a rough evening. I really wanted food badly and became restless and fidgety again in the afternoon – even a little depressed. Can't believe how persistent my inner jerk is at making up nonsense rationalizations.

Despite the emotional tug of war, I have felt surprisingly energetic and have had decent mental clarity. No headaches or anything like that, thank goodness.

This evening after the girls went to bed I blended tomorrow's smoothies. Right now, I'm lying in bed, approximating that I will get about 7 hours of sleep. Another day… no cheats (except for that accidental piece of cereal), and no defeats. Thought that was cool because it rhymed.

JOURNAL, DAY 3

Check in 1 (10am or later)
How many hours of sleep did I get last night? _______________
Did I drink enough water yesterday? _____________________
What am I learning and experiencing?

What are my main concerns and predictions for the day?

Were yesterday's concerns/predictions accurate?

How can I apply what I am learning?

Check in 2 (6pm or later)
Have I succeeded in my daily goals so far?

How I feel so far (Emotionally, physically, relationally, etc):

Problems I have encountered and how I am dealing with them:

What was the most difficult part (or time) of the day?

What can I learn to do differently tomorrow (and in the future) to help me stay on track?

CALEB'S JOURNAL, DAY 3 -

Our lives are full and busy. Because of this, we often don't make time to take life-improving steps. Rather than breaking out of our stagnant environments, we make excuses for staying in them. So, remember: while it may not always be easy to see the virtue in blending up vegetables, it's hard not to see the virtue in breaking out of our excuse-making mentalities. This is the key to a more fulfilling life.

Check in 1: <u>VIDEO</u>

Morning number 3 is off to a good start. I have my smoothies made and my day laid out for me. I went shopping last night because I was low on supplies. Right now, oranges were not very expensive – about $2.99 for a five pound bag, so I bought two bags. You've got to love when you find great deals.

I want to be careful not to just add fruit to my smoothies, because I don't want to be getting too much sugar. Even though it is good sugar, too much of it can be counterproductive overall.

I worked out for about 15 minutes on my Total Gym doing triceps, chest, and abs. That was at about 9 o'clock at night. Normally, I would probably advise people to work out earlier in the day, because I've heard it's better for your body not to get too worked up before sleep. But also, because you burn a lot more calories if you work out in the morning.

However, in my case, and in your case too probably, we have to work it in whenever we can, sticking to the principle that any exercise is better than none. When I'm at home all day with the girls, I'm not guaranteed a break.

For the most part, yesterday was slow and arduous. Emotionally, I dealt with extreme boredom, restlessness, and waves of depression from not getting my comfort foods. So, the fact that I didn't cave in yesterday is a huge success, and I want to make sure to celebrate even the small successes.

I do feel that it becomes easier to say no once you gain a little momentum. And, I believe that day three will be a tad easier, even though I am not over the hump yet.

Check in 2:

Day 3 felt much like my first two days. It started out easy, but got pretty difficult. Very difficult, in fact. My work partner ordered a footlong steak and cheese sub and ate it in front of me (not to be rude, but just because we are together all day).

I'm convinced that there's something about doing a smoothie cleanse that enhances the smell of food. At one point, I actually had to go into Subway to use the bathroom and I was blown away at how drawn in I was by the smells of the spices and meats and vegetables.

I drank my 64 oz of homemade smoothie up before 4pm and found myself needing something more around 6pm. So, with a Jamba juice nearby, I dropped in and ordered an Acia Super-antioxidant smoothie.

By the way, I would caution you to do your homework on the smoothies that you order when you're out, because a lot of these places aren't as selective about the ingredients they use. About a year ago, on one of my failed-smoothie-fast attempts, I discovered that the Acai Super-Antioxidant smoothie had soymilk in it. And, a large scoop of raspberry sherbet. No wonder it tasted so good. It was darn near a milkshake.

Now, when I order it, I have to substitute the sherbet for real raspberries and substitute the soymilk for freshly squeezed orange juice. Taste-wise, it's honestly not even that much different, and if you're needing something, it more than does the trick.

Although I'll be at home tomorrow, I may make a larger amount of smoothie than usual, simply because I don't want to run out and be shorthanded again. My parents will also be in town and I will certainly be tempted to join them when they order pizza or Chinese. I will need something to combat the temptation. Maybe an extra scoop of Chocolate protein mix? Just saying.

Work is almost finished today and I'll be headed home shortly (at least, I hope). While I normally try to squeeze a game or two in on the Xbox once I'm home, I will probably go straight to bed instead. I've found that it's sometimes easier to sleep your hunger away, especially when temptations are at their max

JOURNAL, DAY 4

Check in 1 (10am or later)
How many hours of sleep did I get last night? _______________
Did I drink enough water yesterday? _________________________
What am I learning and experiencing?

What are my main concerns and predictions for the day?

Were yesterday's concerns/predictions accurate?

How can I apply what I am learning?

Check in 2 (6pm or later)
Have I succeeded in my daily goals so far?

How I feel so far (Emotionally, physically, relationally, etc):

Problems I have encountered and how I am dealing with them:

What was the most difficult part (or time) of the day?

What can I learn to do differently tomorrow (and in the future) to help me stay on track?

CALEB'S JOURNAL, DAY 4 -

We seem to be good at finding special occasions – at the start of the day, the end of the day, and in the middle of each day. Stay strong and be smart enough to see these "special occasions" for what they are – excuses that weak people make to avoid doing something hard.

Check in 1: <u>VIDEO</u>

This morning, I felt a little bit light-headed for some reason. I slept for about 7 hours, but it was a bit broken up. So, while I didn't exactly reach my sleep goals, I at least tried. Some days, my schedule makes it hard.

As far as my lightheadedness goes, I think I might actually be a little bit dehydrated, despite all the fluid intake I'm getting. I have a feeling that my body just isn't quite used this yet, and I'll have to be very intentional about drinking even more water than I have been.

I know that while my parents are here it will be difficult to stay away from food, especially because eating out is one of our favorite pastimes. It will be kind of strange not to go out to a restaurant. Or, to go, but not eat. Wish me luck.

Check in 2: <u>VIDEO</u>

I'm not going to lie… today was pretty dang hard. I wanted so badly to join my parents for dinner, eating a delicious smelling rotisserie chicken, corn on the cob, steamed vegetables, and more. Sitting and watching felt like torture!

But, even before that, my day was already difficult – from about noon till 7pm. These were the times when I was seriously rationalizing, trying to figure out how I might be able to eat a piece of chicken without cheating.

At one point, I had a sort of panicky moment and felt trapped. It was as though it suddenly dawned on me how many more days I still had to go and wondered how on earth I'd make it. Luckily, that moment passed pretty quickly though.

One thing that helps me stay motivated is the fact that I truly do believe my body has suffered some serious damage over the years and that my diet has been the cause of it. I normally only get this realization when I'm recovering from a junk food hangover and for a few fleeting moments (before coma sets in), I get inspired to change things. Unfortunately for me, those moments have always passed pretty quickly as well. At least I'm being proactive now.

JOURNAL, DAY 5

Check in 1 (10am or later)

How many hours of sleep did I get last night? _______________

Did I drink enough water yesterday? _________________________

What am I learning and experiencing?

What are my main concerns and predictions for the day?

Were yesterday's concerns/predictions accurate?

How can I apply what I am learning?

Check in 2 (6pm or later)

Have I succeeded in my daily goals so far?

How I feel so far (Emotionally, physically, relationally, etc):

Problems I have encountered and how I am dealing with them:

What was the most difficult part (or time) of the day?

What can I learn to do differently tomorrow (and in the future) to help me stay on track?

CALEB'S JOURNAL, DAY 5 -

DAILY INSPIRATION:

I often see people who are in great shape, and I think, "Man, I would love to look like that." It's as though I assume they have some advantage over me that doesn't require them to strive and labor for what they have. This perspective does an injustice – not just to them, but to myself as well. Because, if I think they don't have to work hard for success, I won't think that I'll have to work hard for it either. What sets most successful people apart isn't luck, but the commitment to work hard. In a way, this is good news and bad news. Bad, because it means that our excuses are no good. Good, because it means that a better life is possible, just a little discomfort away!

Check in 1: <u>VIDEO</u>

This morning was pretty rough again, much like yesterday. I woke up feeling unenergized, light-headed, and wishing I could just keep sleeping. This only leads me further to believe that I must not be getting enough water.

Last night was crazy difficult, I'm not going to lie. The hardest part of my day was probably at dinner time (roughly 6pm), and it lasted until I went to bed. My smoothies just weren't enticing at all. It felt like I was chugging green slime while everybody else was feasting away. But, I can't say that I didn't predict moments like this would happen.

While there have been some obvious downsides to this plan, I must say that I haven't noticed any arthritis in my feet lately, and that my focus seems to have improved. I guess I'll see how things improve as time goes on.

Check in 2: <u>VIDEO</u>

This was probably my best evening since I started. For the first time, I felt pretty darn good. Good enough to take my daughters on a walk around the lake… twice! That equals just over 4 miles total. When I got back, I worked out for a bit on the Total Gym, doing some work on my abs, pecs, and lats.

The nauseousness and lack of energy that I felt earlier are now gone! I even had a few moments of clarity when it seemed like the neurons in my brain were being "dusted off" so to speak. It felt like my memory was working better than usual as well.

I ended up having to make more smoothie when I got home, as I was low on energy after my walk/workout. I blended up a tad more and then drank down my dinner. I've got tomorrow's smoothies already blended and stored in the fridge, so I'll be in bed soon, ready to face tomorrow!

JOURNAL, DAY 6

Check in 1 (10am or later)
How many hours of sleep did I get last night? _______________
Did I drink enough water yesterday? _________________________
What am I learning and experiencing?

What are my main concerns and predictions for the day?

Were yesterday's concerns/predictions accurate?

How can I apply what I am learning?

Check in 2 (6pm or later)
Have I succeeded in my daily goals so far?

How I feel so far (Emotionally, physically, relationally, etc):

Problems I have encountered and how I am dealing with them:

What was the most difficult part (or time) of the day?

What can I learn to do differently tomorrow (and in the future) to help me stay on track?

CALEB'S JOURNAL, DAY 6 -

One of the most common lies we tell ourselves is that we'll start tomorrow. Tomorrow, we'll begin to eat healthy. Tomorrow, we'll start going to the gym. Tomorrow, we'll start the hard work of changing. One way to overcome this tempting lie is to realize that tomorrow, things won't be any easier. In fact, whatever is difficult now may only be more difficult later. Don't let any more of your life slip through your fingertips by believing this lie!

Check in 1:

This morning, I woke up late and had to scramble out the door to be on time for work. I almost forgot to bring the smoothies I made last night. That would have been unfortunate. But, I suppose the good thing about being in a hurry is that you don't have time to think about how you're feeling.

Once I was on the road and had time to think about it, I noticed that I had a slight headache. Not a bad one. In fact, I felt pretty energetic. So, once I made it to work, I decided to take advantage of that extra energy by doing 30 squats before punching in. Nice to feel like I have already begun to meet my light-exercise quota.

I've been drinking water that is distilled because I've heard that it is good for cleansing periods such as this. As I understand it, normal water has minerals, but distilled water has none, which means that it is looking for minerals to bind to. So, when you drink it, it clings to excess minerals in your body and helps filter them out. That is my unscientific explanation, anyway. Don't quote me on it.

Check in 2:

While being slightly easier than the last few days, tonight wasn't exactly a breeze. Right when I've started to think that my work partner is a really nice guy, he goes and orders a steak burrito and eats it right in front of me. Jerk. All I had was some green slush to slurp on. Not so tasty, but, let's see... it's only pure liquid vitamins! When I outlive him, it looks like I'll get the last laugh!

Seriously though, I feel like this is all starting to get a little easier, if only because I've gotten better at saying no to everything I love. I'm not gonna fib to you... the first time I drove past my favorite restaurant without stopping in, it felt like a part of me had died. Now though, it feels like I've begun to slow down some of that negative momentum that has slowly been killing me.

The hardest part of my day today was at 2pm. Not sure why. The best part of my day was around noon. Also, not sure why. For whatever reason, I felt great all throughout the morning. My brain was functioning like a well-oiled machine and I wasn't fighting any fatigue.

I've been drinking from a gallon of distilled water that I bought earlier and have already almost finished the entire thing. I feel confident that it will be gone before bedtime. Also, I've done quite quite a few squats since this morning. All in all, this day is going pretty well.

JOURNAL, DAY 7

Check in 1 (10am or later)
How many hours of sleep did I get last night? _______________
Did I drink enough water yesterday? _________________________
What am I learning and experiencing?

What are my main concerns and predictions for the day?

Were yesterday's concerns/predictions accurate?

How can I apply what I am learning?

Check in 2 (6pm or later)
Have I succeeded in my daily goals so far?

How I feel so far (Emotionally, physically, relationally, etc):

Problems I have encountered and how I am dealing with them:

What was the most difficult part (or time) of the day?

What can I learn to do differently tomorrow (and in the future) to help me stay on track?

CALEB'S JOURNAL, DAY 7 -

DAILY INSPIRATION:

If ever you find yourself sitting there, staring at your favorite dishes and wondering why on earth you're not diving in, remember that the immediate comfort of food is short-lived, but the effects of healthy living are long-lasting. It's true that nothing tastes as good as being healthy feels!

Check in 1:

Today started out wonderfully. I woke up early and couldn't go back to bed. I couldn't figure out why, and then it finally clicked… I was rested. That's why I couldn't sleep! Don't you see? This is a great sign! Children wake up at the crack of dawn while their parents are still praying for five more minutes, because children actually feel rested. We adults rarely do! I believe that my energetic early-rise may be a sign that I am beginning to achieve some of my goals.

But, since I spent the night at my parents' house, it means that my smoothie-making equipment isn't accessible. Fortunately, my brother left a Vitamix blender here, which will allow me to make my daily dose with the fruit and vegetables from my parents' fridge.

I've already hit the rowing machine this morning, rowing over 1000 meters. That makes: a bit of light exercise, some water, and a couple thermoses full of liquid vitamins. I am right on track! Day number seven, let's go!

Check in 2: <u>VIDEO</u>

We spent the day at Brookfield Zoo. It was a good day, and we did a lot of walking. My mom's fitbit counted 17,000 steps, which I believe equates to over a few miles in distance. At the end of it all, I felt ready for a break, but still pretty good.

Things got a little tougher afterwards when everyone decided to go to Wendy', ordering burgers and fries and devouring it in front of me. I cried an inner tear or two, trying to live vicariously through everyone else's taste buds.

The temptation soon passed, however, and once it was gone, I already felt very glad that I had remained strong. In fact, it wasn't long before they were envying me – for my willpower, but also, for the high amount of energy I had compared to them.

Still going strong. I am almost a third of the way finished, and I can officially say… it does get easier over time.

JOURNAL, DAY 8

Check in 1 (10am or later)
How many hours of sleep did I get last night? _______________
Did I drink enough water yesterday? _______________________
What am I learning and experiencing?

What are my main concerns and predictions for the day?

Were yesterday's concerns/predictions accurate?

How can I apply what I am learning?

Check in 2 (6pm or later)
Have I succeeded in my daily goals so far?

How I feel so far (Emotionally, physically, relationally, etc):

Problems I have encountered and how I am dealing with them:

What was the most difficult part (or time) of the day?

What can I learn to do differently tomorrow (and in the future) to help me stay on track?

CALEB'S JOURNAL, DAY 8 -

DAILY INSPIRATION:

Comfort is just a bandaid. When you take an aspirin for a headache, your headache doesn't really go away. Your senses just become temporarily numb to the pain. The same is true for emotional pain. When we feel depressed from not being able to eat whatever we want, it is because the numbing effect of our comfort foods has worn off, and now, we are facing whichever tough emotions we are accustomed to burying. When you feel it, don't see it as a sign that this plan isn't working. Instead, see it as a sign that your senses are returning and you are slowly becoming healthier.

Check in 1:

Despite all the miles I walked yesterday and my small bit of exercise on the rowing machine, I was unpleasantly surprised to see that my weight hadn't changed since yesterday. Really? Come on! It's kind of discouraging and frustrating. I don't know the reason for this. Maybe it's just one of those plateaus people seem to run into on their way to their goals.

Check in 2:

So far, the hardest part of my day was around 3pm. It lasted till about 6 p.m. My work partner, as always, ordered a footlong Potbelly sub and ate it in front of me. I have to admit, I enjoy even the smell. Somehow, the smell of food is actually a bit of comfort when I know I won't be tasting it.

On another note, I can feel the weight loss affecting my entire body. I feel like my joints suffer less resistance from normal movements, and I feel that even my shirt feels a little looser around the belly area. This is encouraging.

I also feel like my memory is improving. I don't have to think quite as long to find the words I'm looking for and I seem to be quicker at recalling events from yesterday. This is encouraging as well.

I am starting to feel really glad that I did all of this and that I have been faithful to my commitment thus far. While I know I still have a long ways to go, I'm getting excited about the remainder of the journey.

JOURNAL, DAY 9

Check in 1 (10am or later)
How many hours of sleep did I get last night? _______________
Did I drink enough water yesterday? ___________________________
What am I learning and experiencing?

What are my main concerns and predictions for the day?

Were yesterday's concerns/predictions accurate?

How can I apply what I am learning?

Check in 2 (6pm or later)
Have I succeeded in my daily goals so far?

How I feel so far (Emotionally, physically, relationally, etc):

Problems I have encountered and how I am dealing with them:

What was the most difficult part (or time) of the day?

What can I learn to do differently tomorrow (and in the future) to help me stay on track?

CALEB'S JOURNAL, DAY 9 -

DAILY INSPIRATION:

As I get better at resisting my impulses, I realize that my willpower is growing and that it is affecting me – not just with food, but in all areas of life. For example, when somebody says something offensive to me and I'm tempted to get defensive, I react much more calmly. Being disciplined in one area, I find, makes me disciplined in most other areas as well.

Check in 1:

Day nine has been hard, but not because of the smoothie plan. Rather, because of all the normal life mixed in with it. For a number of reasons, it has just been a bit difficult to juggle all the various balls of life today.

All morning, my daughters were both crying. It's been one of those days. I've felt like the main character of some family sitcom with both of them going nuts while I was trying to get things ready. All in all though, we somehow survived.

Check in 2:

As I check in again, I must say that the most challenging part of my day was when I met up with a friend to watch a movie. We met at the theater like we normally do, only unlike past times, I did not order a burger and a beer this time. It felt strange and made me miss food. A lot.

Still, the momentum is going and I plan to keep it going. I will now try to begin to focus more on my sleep, as well as my water intake. Reclaiming my life one day at a time. It comes slowly but surely.

JOURNAL, DAY 10

Check in 1 (10am or later)

How many hours of sleep did I get last night? _______________

Did I drink enough water yesterday? _________________________

What am I learning and experiencing?

What are my main concerns and predictions for the day?

Were yesterday's concerns/predictions accurate?

How can I apply what I am learning?

Check in 2 (6pm or later)

Have I succeeded in my daily goals so far?

How I feel so far (Emotionally, physically, relationally, etc):

Problems I have encountered and how I am dealing with them:

What was the most difficult part (or time) of the day?

What can I learn to do differently tomorrow (and in the future) to help me stay on track?

CALEB'S JOURNAL, DAY 10 -

DAILY INSPIRATION:

It's always hard to resist the temptation to eat unhealthy foods. However, nearly every time you do, you regret it within minutes. Junk food appears satisfying, but it's actually not. Five minutes later, you usually feel it taking its toll on your levels of energy and mental clarity. So, try to think of this thirty day period as one piece of time that you'll have the rest of your life not to regret.

Check in 1:

Day ten was another success. I'm proud that I stuck to my guns last night, despite the many temptations that I found myself in the midst of while I was out at the theatre. I shudder to think that it could have all ended there!

This morning, I weighed exactly 195 lbs. This felt good, because, in the last few days, I have not seen the results I have been hoping for. Finally, there is some evidence that my weight is still continuing to drop.

I got about 6-7 hours of sleep last night, broken up a bit by my daughter who woke up at 4am from a bad dream. I went into her room and slept by her on the floor for about twenty minutes until she fell asleep again. Then, I went back to my own bed. It was actually a precious moment.

Today, I feel pretty well for the most part. My skin seems to look better too. Also, I've noticed that my stomach, overall, seems less bloated. I don't know which foods in particular I am sensitive to, but in past few years, my stomach seems to have started taking more time to digest food. Maybe some of this is just a natural part of aging. Even still, I can't help but suspect that it has to do with all the fake stuff we put in our foods. Just a theory.

Check in 2:

I don't have a lot to add to the journal tonight. Perhaps only that I am seeing how difficult real life changes are to make. Also, I'm seeing that the right changes are worth making. Results aren't seen right away. They take time. For that, it is important to have patience with the process.

JOURNAL, DAY 11

Check in 1 (10am or later)
How many hours of sleep did I get last night? _______________
Did I drink enough water yesterday? _________________________
What am I learning and experiencing?

What are my main concerns and predictions for the day?

Were yesterday's concerns/predictions accurate?

How can I apply what I am learning?

Check in 2 (6pm or later)
Have I succeeded in my daily goals so far?

How I feel so far (Emotionally, physically, relationally, etc):

Problems I have encountered and how I am dealing with them:

What was the most difficult part (or time) of the day?

What can I learn to do differently tomorrow (and in the future) to help me stay on track?

CALEB'S JOURNAL, DAY 11 -

DAILY INSPIRATION:

Remember that those people who don't understand your health goals or who may even be teasing you now are probably the same people who, later on, upon seeing the remarkable changes in you, will be asking to know your secret.

Check in 1:

This morning was easy. I didn't even feel hungry until noon. I did a light workout this morning on the Total Gym and did some stretching as well. You've got to be thankful for the easier moments!

Check in 2:

My dad came into town, which was nice. Though it is always nice to see him, it means temptations will probably be high yet again. Sure enough, he ordered an Italian sub. I got free smells. This took place at about 2pm and it was probably the hardest part of my day.

On a positive note, I've begun to feel more satisfied by my smoothies. When I first started this whole thing, they did nothing for my hunger. Now, my body seems to be getting more sensitive and I actually feel filled up when I drink them.

All things considered, I feel pretty decent. I have only had very few traces of arthritis pain. I believe this is due to the decrease of inflammation causing foods. It's good to keep those positive changes in focus because it helps me stay strong.

JOURNAL, DAY 12

Check in 1 (10am or later)
How many hours of sleep did I get last night? ________________
Did I drink enough water yesterday? ____________________
What am I learning and experiencing?

What are my main concerns and predictions for the day?

Were yesterday's concerns/predictions accurate?

How can I apply what I am learning?

Check in 2 (6pm or later)
Have I succeeded in my daily goals so far?

How I feel so far (Emotionally, physically, relationally, etc):

Problems I have encountered and how I am dealing with them:

What was the most difficult part (or time) of the day?

What can I learn to do differently tomorrow (and in the future) to help me stay on track?

CALEB'S JOURNAL, DAY 12 -

DAILY INSPIRATION:

It has been said, "Those who don't make time for health must make time for sickness." While eating right may seem like a luxury, it actually is not. And, it is better to do it because you chose to, rather than because an illness forced you to.

Check in 1: <u>VIDEO</u>

This morning was a bit of a rocky ride. I was up late last night tiling in the basement and felt too tired to hit the blender. So, now I am at the mercy of Jamba Juice again, which will be expensive, but better than having nothing.

I ordered my Acai Super-antioxidant again, subbing the raspberry sherbet for real raspberries, the soymilk for freshly squeezed orange juice, and the vitamin packet for 3G energy boost (whatever that is). It turned out to be great and just what I needed to feel energized.

This morning, I was a bit disappointed to see that my weight had actually gone up. I wonder if I'm doing something wrong, because I'm not losing the amount of weight that I thought I would. I'm guessing that this is because A. I am not getting enough sleep and exercise along with my smoothies, or B. I am adding too much sugar, and I may need to tone it down. Or, it could be both. I wonder if I should adjust my plan. I'll keep this in consideration in the following days.

Check in 2:

Tonight, in a sense, I fell off the wagon. I ate a piece of peppermint candy from a dish on the desk at work. Now, this may not sound like a big deal, but it actually made me feel discouraged. I think it is because I am somewhat of an all-or-nothing person.

Yet, I know that all-or-nothing thinking isn't good, because it usually keeps us from giving anything when we can't give our all. Anyway, I'm not going to let this small mistake get me down.

JOURNAL, DAY 13

Check in 1 (10am or later)

How many hours of sleep did I get last night? _______________

Did I drink enough water yesterday? _________________________

What am I learning and experiencing?

What are my main concerns and predictions for the day?

Were yesterday's concerns/predictions accurate?

How can I apply what I am learning?

Check in 2 (6pm or later)

Have I succeeded in my daily goals so far?

How I feel so far (Emotionally, physically, relationally, etc):

Problems I have encountered and how I am dealing with them:

What was the most difficult part (or time) of the day?

What can I learn to do differently tomorrow (and in the future) to help me stay on track?

CALEB'S JOURNAL, DAY 13 -

DAILY INSPIRATION:

We tend to blame the solutions instead of the problems. When we try something and it doesn't work, our first instinct is to say, "So much for that idea." But, it usually wasn't the solution that was faulty, it was our application of it. At some point, we didn't do it right or we didn't do it long enough. Just because something hasn't worked for you in the past, don't rule it out as ineffective. Remember that consistency and diligence are required to make this (or any) plan work!

Check in 1:

Wow, this morning was chaotic. Getting out the door for church was not without drama. My wife and I had a "heated talk," as we'll call it, and the outcome was a brief cooldown period away from each other before coming back to make up. How's that for real life?

In the realness of it all, I missed my chance to blend and ended up unprepared for the day. My stomach started to grumble and I ended up ordering a mango-pineapple smoothie from Mcdonalds. Now, I don't know if anything in it is real – the mangos or the pineapple. I just know that the sugar is, and there is a lot of it. Oh well. Desperate times call for desperate measures.

Check in 2:

Later on at home, I was able to blend a full 8-cup portion for the afternoon and evening. I felt a bit tired for some reason, but I think I know why... I was crashing from that Mcdonald's sugar-rush from earlier.

While I was at the store picking up some produce for the coming week, I took a gander through some of the aisles and it all got me thinking. I know will soon be back to eating food again, but I don't want to go back to my old patterns. Some of them were just compulsive and destructive. I think that if I kept on living the way I was, my lifespan would be drastically shortened.

Anyway, all this to say that I want to keep some of the changes I've made. Short-lived phases do nothing in the long run. I need real, lasting changes. I need moderation and consistency to be constant fixtures in my life. I plan on using my remaining 17 days to start figuring out how.

JOURNAL, DAY 14

Check in 1 (10am or later)
How many hours of sleep did I get last night? ________________
Did I drink enough water yesterday? _____________________
What am I learning and experiencing?

What are my main concerns and predictions for the day?

Were yesterday's concerns/predictions accurate?

How can I apply what I am learning?

Check in 2 (6pm or later)
Have I succeeded in my daily goals so far?

How I feel so far (Emotionally, physically, relationally, etc):

Problems I have encountered and how I am dealing with them:

What was the most difficult part (or time) of the day?

What can I learn to do differently tomorrow (and in the future) to help me stay on track?

CALEB'S JOURNAL, DAY 14 -

Check in 1:

This morning, I woke up tired, probably because I only got about 6 hours of sleep. The sad truth is that I'm still actually getting more sleep than I usually do. Some lifestyle changes are really hard to make because of the many variables outside of our control.

I'm doing well though as far as staying away from food. I made a few smoothies today that lasted me while I was at work. I believe they were pretty nutritious, however, they weren't the best tasting. I may have overdone it with the amount of spinach I used.

Check in 2:

It was a bit difficult tonight to stay away from food. For some reason, Subway is tempting me more than any other place. I fantasize about a footlong spicy Italian and all the fixings I normally put on it. Oh man. I have to stop talking about it.

Most people that I talk to want to know more about what I'm doing. Some think I'm crazy. Others wish they had the discipline to do it themselves and say that they know they need to. I tell them that I didn't have the discipline either. In fact, my lack of discipline was hard on my body, which is why I needed to do something.

Tomorrow marks my halfway point. I can't believe I made it this far. It has been a pretty cool experience. I sense that I am growing – not just in my discipline towards food, but in all other areas. I am simply becoming a stronger person. I am becoming clearer about my goals and about why I am after them. This helps me to pursue them more wholeheartedly.

JOURNAL, DAY 15

Check in 1 (10am or later)
How many hours of sleep did I get last night? _______________
Did I drink enough water yesterday? ____________________
What am I learning and experiencing?

What are my main concerns and predictions for the day?

Were yesterday's concerns/predictions accurate?

How can I apply what I am learning?

Check in 2 (6pm or later)
Have I succeeded in my daily goals so far?

How I feel so far (Emotionally, physically, relationally, etc):

Problems I have encountered and how I am dealing with them:

What was the most difficult part (or time) of the day?

What can I learn to do differently tomorrow (and in the future) to help me stay on track?

CALEB'S JOURNAL, DAY 15 -

There is a certain type of pleasure and satisfaction that come from setting, having, and reaching our goals. Often though, we aren't really aiming for a specific target. This plan gives us a specific target, as well as a chance to experience that sense of fulfillment that comes from hitting it.

Check in 1:

Holy cow… I am officially at the halfway point! I remember day two when I didn't think I'd ever make it here, blinded by the agony of losing so many comforts. Now, just look at me… feeling good, looking better, weighing less. Has it been worth it? For sure!

Check in 2:

I think I forgot to mention that at my weigh-in this morning, I was at 192.4 lbs. I feel like I'm hitting another plateau. I suppose it could be that my water intake hasn't been as good lately, which affects how well my body rids of excess.

I suppose that the hardest part of my day was around 8pm when my wife whipped up a huge bowl of macaroni and cheese for herself and the kids. Oh man… mac and cheese is a major weakness of mine! Where is my inspiration? Don't leave me now!

Fortunately, I made it through the hardest parts without budging. Day 15, in the can. All in all, I'm still feeling pretty good. I'm officially halfway there and excited about the remainder of my journey!

JOURNAL, DAY 16

Check in 1 (10am or later)
How many hours of sleep did I get last night? _______________
Did I drink enough water yesterday? _____________________
What am I learning and experiencing?

What are my main concerns and predictions for the day?

Were yesterday's concerns/predictions accurate?

How can I apply what I am learning?

Check in 2 (6pm or later)
Have I succeeded in my daily goals so far?

How I feel so far (Emotionally, physically, relationally, etc):

Problems I have encountered and how I am dealing with them:

What was the most difficult part (or time) of the day?

What can I learn to do differently tomorrow (and in the future) to help me stay on track?

CALEB'S JOURNAL, DAY 16 -

DAILY INSPIRATION:

Sometimes, it takes getting what you want in order to know that it's not what you wanted. When you get the mental fog from eating a donut, you quickly realize that it's not what you wanted. Yet, when you get the rush of a natural high, you realize that it is what you wanted, whether you knew it or not. Be smart enough to realize what you really want, or your impulses will do your deciding for you.

Check in 1:

Today, I drove off today in a hurry, not remembering the smoothies I had prepared last night. Rats. I was so proud too... for being so strong and organized yesterday, despite all the temptation around me. Oh well.

One thing I want to reiterate (which I think can't be said enough), is the fact that you don't see immediate results on this plan. It takes quite a while (and quite a few days of feeling miserable) before you start to feel better. In health goals (and perhaps, in all areas of life), shortsightedness is a serious roadblock. No one will ever make it past day two without big-picture vision.

Today, I noticed that I had a lot of energy. I used it to do exercise throughout the day, looking for opportunities to do squats and pushups anywhere I could. Normally, such things would quickly get me fatigued and short of breath. Today though, I felt energized by it, as though I couldn't get enough.

I just keep thinking that, if not for this commitment, I would never have experienced this type of energy, and I'm becoming very determined not to go back to where I was, because that lifestyle is painful. You always feel drained and exhausted. You always feel like life is a blur, and like you're not really mentally present. This is better, no doubt. As they say, "Nothing tastes as good as being healthy feels."

Check in 2:

So, you know that I forgot the smoothies I made at home, right? No problem. I decided that I would save those for tomorrow and rely on Jamba Juice today. Yeah, it's expensive, and yeah, a tad on the sugary side, but this isn't about perfection. It's about doing what you can with what you have.

JOURNAL, DAY 17

Check in 1 (10am or later)

How many hours of sleep did I get last night? _______________

Did I drink enough water yesterday? ___________________________

What am I learning and experiencing?

What are my main concerns and predictions for the day?

Were yesterday's concerns/predictions accurate?

How can I apply what I am learning?

Check in 2 (6pm or later)

Have I succeeded in my daily goals so far?

How I feel so far (Emotionally, physically, relationally, etc):

Problems I have encountered and how I am dealing with them:

What was the most difficult part (or time) of the day?

What can I learn to do differently tomorrow (and in the future) to help me stay on track?

CALEB'S JOURNAL, DAY 17 -

Sometimes, we don't want to look at our goals because we know deep down that our actions are not in line with them. It takes courage to break the pattern of rationalization. But, this is the path toward improvement. Rise above your emotions. Try to realize that they aren't always telling you the truth.

Check in 1:

This morning, I woke up and felt ready to go. My smoothies were already made from two days ago and were sitting in thermoses in my fridge. Yesterday's inconvenience is today's advantage.

I got on the scale and was surprised again that my weight still hadn't changed. Maybe this is why I've heard it said that you shouldn't check your weight every day. It can be a bit deceiving.

Other than that, I feel pretty good though for the most part. I just need to remember to drink more water because that's something that doesn't always come natural for me.

Check in 2:

My dad was in town today to help me out in the basement, and as usual, it was hard not to join in the eating of pizza and other snacks. I keep having to remind myself that this plan wouldn't go on forever. It was as though my tastebuds needed reassurance that someday, they would have a happy reunion with their long-lost fattening friends.

Other than that, there isn't a whole lot to say about today. Day 17 is just about done. After today, there are only 12 more days to go. The finish line is in sight!

JOURNAL, DAY 18

Check in 1 (10am or later)

How many hours of sleep did I get last night? _______________

Did I drink enough water yesterday? _____________________

What am I learning and experiencing?

What are my main concerns and predictions for the day?

Were yesterday's concerns/predictions accurate?

How can I apply what I am learning?

Check in 2 (6pm or later)

Have I succeeded in my daily goals so far?

How I feel so far (Emotionally, physically, relationally, etc):

Problems I have encountered and how I am dealing with them:

What was the most difficult part (or time) of the day?

What can I learn to do differently tomorrow (and in the future) to help me stay on track?

CALEB'S JOURNAL, DAY 18 -

Check in 1:

This morning seemed to start out badly. I was Moody. Also, I was trapped inside, being that I was on dad-duty. Not that it's something I don't enjoy, it's just that I sometimes get cabin fever when I'm stuck in one place for too long.

One redeeming factor was that my smoothies tasted delicious. And, I finally broke the 190 barrier and weighed in at 189 pounds this morning. It feels good to be making some measurable progress. And, apart from the moodiness I feel, there are some ways I actually feel better. My breathing is easier and I have more energy.

Check in 2:

Later on in the day I had to go for a drive because I was feeling like I was going crazy. I went to True Value Hardware and bought some stuff for a project that I'm working on in the basement. It felt good just to get out of the house.

I'm at day 18 and it is almost over. Right now, I'm laying down to go to bed. It's been a rough day, but it hasn't conquered me. I'm over the hump now and I can safely say that I'm ready for the downhill ride. Good night all. Hoping for an energetic, positive day tomorrow.

JOURNAL, DAY 19

Check in 1 (10am or later)
How many hours of sleep did I get last night? ________________
Did I drink enough water yesterday? ____________________
What am I learning and experiencing?

What are my main concerns and predictions for the day?

Were yesterday's concerns/predictions accurate?

How can I apply what I am learning?

Check in 2 (6pm or later)
Have I succeeded in my daily goals so far?

How I feel so far (Emotionally, physically, relationally, etc):

Problems I have encountered and how I am dealing with them:

What was the most difficult part (or time) of the day?

What can I learn to do differently tomorrow (and in the future) to help me stay on track?

CALEB'S JOURNAL, DAY 19 -

Be grateful for those times when this process hurts, because those are the times when you can do the most growing. At no other time are you so exposed to your weakness. At no other time will you find such a great opportunity to master it!

Check in 1:

Last night I got about six hours of sleep. As usual, it was less than ideal, but it seems to be my norm.

My weight hasn't gone down since yesterday, even though on a long-term scale it is headed steadily downward. My target is to be in the lower 170s. Partially, because I would like to run in a marathon, and I feel that weighing less would be less stressful on my joints.

I feel pretty good overall. I've had a few strange moments when I have felt angry for no apparent reasons. It may or may not have to do with my recent lifestyle changes, although I'm not one hundred percent sure. It's hard to say. Hopefully, it is a sign that I'm on the path of healing – emotionally, physically, and mentally.

Check in 2:

Today has been difficult. Strange emotions have continued to flood through me. However, I've managed to deal with them by staying busy – one of the best cures for anxiety and depression!

I have been satisfied with my smoothies for the most part, except perhaps for a few moments during the afternoon when tacos sounded really, really good. Oh well. I'll have to save that desire for another time.

In the busyness of life, I have neglected my exercise to some degree and hope to get back on track in the coming days. It hasn't helped that my Total Gym has been temporarily stored away, due to a project that I'm working on in the basement.

JOURNAL, DAY 20

Check in 1 (10am or later)

How many hours of sleep did I get last night? _______________

Did I drink enough water yesterday? _________________________

What am I learning and experiencing?

What are my main concerns and predictions for the day?

Were yesterday's concerns/predictions accurate?

How can I apply what I am learning?

Check in 2 (6pm or later)

Have I succeeded in my daily goals so far?

How I feel so far (Emotionally, physically, relationally, etc):

Problems I have encountered and how I am dealing with them:

What was the most difficult part (or time) of the day?

What can I learn to do differently tomorrow (and in the future) to help me stay on track?

CALEB'S JOURNAL, DAY 20 -

When you feel good naturally, you are less in need of unnatural ways to feel good. When you are getting enough water, sleep, vitamins, and nutrients, your desires decrease for all those fake, unhealthy pick-me-ups.

Check in 1: <u>VIDEO</u>

Today, I am working a full 24 hour shift. These longer workdays are more difficult to plan for. Especially when my decision to take the shift was last-minute… my boss called me late last night and asked if I could do it. Reluctantly, I said yes.

For whatever reason, my smoothies haven't been very satisfying today. I seem to have gotten my proportions wrong and the taste of spinach is a bit overpowering. My chocolate protein mix has done little to redeem it.

Before work, I weighed in at 189.2 pounds. The changes are small, but visible. I'm learning that on a day-to-day basis, it's probably best not to dwell on slow progress. Instead, dwell on the fact that I'm taking positive actions. This is true no matter how visible the results are.

Check in 2:

Work is always difficult, especially on those days when everyone around me is eating fried chicken. Some of them wave it in front of my face to make me jealous. I tell them that they'll be the envious ones when all this is over.

I managed to choke down the rest of my less-than-delicious smoothie and found resolve to keep plugging away.

JOURNAL, DAY 21

Check in 1 (10am or later)

How many hours of sleep did I get last night? _______________

Did I drink enough water yesterday? _____________________

What am I learning and experiencing?

What are my main concerns and predictions for the day?

Were yesterday's concerns/predictions accurate?

How can I apply what I am learning?

Check in 2 (6pm or later)

Have I succeeded in my daily goals so far?

How I feel so far (Emotionally, physically, relationally, etc):

Problems I have encountered and how I am dealing with them:

What was the most difficult part (or time) of the day?

What can I learn to do differently tomorrow (and in the future) to help me stay on track?

CALEB'S JOURNAL, DAY 21 -

DAILY INSPIRATION:

Remember that there is no such thing as a perfect moment. Waiting to make great life changes is all about the present moment. Take pride in the fact that you are doing something now!

Check in 1:

Today, I weighed in at 188.4 pounds. There's definitely some progress being made. I briefly celebrate each small success and continue on towards my goal.

Once again, I found myself drinking a McDonald's smoothie. Once again, there was so much sugar in it. I could feel it instantly. I guess it's just part of finishing up a 24 hour shift. When your shift ends at 6am, you walk into the day without any preparation for it.

Check in 2:

After getting home to my Vitamix, I was finally able to blend up today's supply. Better yet, I was finally no longer at the mercy of Mcdonald's.

For some reason, I thought I was on day 20, but I'm actually on day 21. It's amazing how time is going by. Especially when some of these moments feel like an eternity.

My light exercise today was softball. It was the church team's first practice. Afterwards, I took my daughter on a two-mile walk around the lake. I guess you could say I'm getting a decent amount of light exercise.

Sleep still seems to be my biggest area of compromise. This is especially true when my job interferes with my regular routine. It is what it is. I just have to make do with what I have.

JOURNAL, DAY 22

Check in 1 (10am or later)
How many hours of sleep did I get last night? _______________
Did I drink enough water yesterday? _________________________
What am I learning and experiencing?

What are my main concerns and predictions for the day?

Were yesterday's concerns/predictions accurate?

How can I apply what I am learning?

Check in 2 (6pm or later)
Have I succeeded in my daily goals so far?

How I feel so far (Emotionally, physically, relationally, etc):

Problems I have encountered and how I am dealing with them:

What was the most difficult part (or time) of the day?

What can I learn to do differently tomorrow (and in the future) to help me stay on track?

CALEB'S JOURNAL, DAY 22 -

Remember the common cliche, "No pain, no gain." The stuff that's easy isn't the stuff that makes us grow. When things become difficult, see it as a measurement of how much you are growing.

Check in 1:

Last night, I got about 6 ½ hours of sleep. This morning, I weighed in at 189.2 lbs. Things continue to head in the right direction, though I still can't help but wish they moved at a quicker pace.

One unfortunate part of my morning was that I wasn't able to make my smoothies, being that my family was still sleeping and I didn't want to wake them with a noisy blender to wake them. So, I relied on Jamba juice this morning.

Around lunchtime, there were no Jamba Juices nearby and I had to rely on Mcdonald's again. I hate doing this, but I sometimes can't think of any other options. Each time this happens, I can literally feel the sugar rushing through me – first, giving me a burst of energy, followed by a sudden crash. It is counterproductive to my health/weight-loss plans.

Despite the less-than ideal circumstances, I feel pretty good overall. My muscles feel sore from yesterday's softball practice, but it's the good kind of sore – the kind that comes from working out.

Check in 2: After 6pm.

Throughout the day I have been more tempted than usual to eat fast food. I believe it's due to the Mcdonald's smoothie I had. Honestly... I think all of that sugar awakens cravings that I haven't been feeling.

I've also done a poor job at staying hydrated throughout the day. When you get off to a bad start, it's easy to feel discouraged. Perhaps there is a lesson to be learned here – an all-or-nothing perspective is hazardous... even when you're more than ⅔ into the journey.

I suppose my advice is that not every day will go as you hope. In fact, most days are full of ups and downs. Some days, those lows can seem drastic. Sometimes, the best thing you can do is accept them as inevitable parts of the journey.

JOURNAL, DAY 23

Check in 1 (10am or later)

How many hours of sleep did I get last night? _______________

Did I drink enough water yesterday? _________________________

What am I learning and experiencing?

What are my main concerns and predictions for the day?

Were yesterday's concerns/predictions accurate?

How can I apply what I am learning?

Check in 2 (6pm or later)

Have I succeeded in my daily goals so far?

How I feel so far (Emotionally, physically, relationally, etc):

Problems I have encountered and how I am dealing with them:

What was the most difficult part (or time) of the day?

What can I learn to do differently tomorrow (and in the future) to help me stay on track?

CALEB'S JOURNAL, DAY 23 -

Check in 1:

Today, I weighed in at 191.2 lbs. Are you serious? Come on! How can I possibly weigh more than I did yesterday? Maybe it has to do with fluid retention. Who knows. Two hours from now, my weight could already be different.

Last night, I slept for about 5 hours. I feel a bit frustrated by this. But, all of these frustrations make me want to be even more conscious about the amount of sugar in my smoothies and to keep myself from having to rely on fast-food smoothies so often.

Today, I am on dad duty again. Also, I'll be meeting with someone from church at 1pm, and I have my first softball game this evening. I'm excited to play – both for the social and physical aspects of it. I believe they are crucial components to a healthy lifestyle.

Check in 2:

This evening went as follows:
Light exercise - check!
Plenty of water - check!
Stayed away from food? Check!
Was it crazily difficult? Check!

Tonight after my first softball game (which we tied by the way), I tried out some of my new camping gear (pie irons, which you can make all sorts of goodies with). I cooked a few campfire pizzas for my wife and daughter and sat back while they ate, doing my best to get filled on sights and smells. Somehow, I managed. Day 23, done. I'm one step closer to my goal!

JOURNAL, DAY 24

Check in 1 (10am or later)
How many hours of sleep did I get last night? _______________
Did I drink enough water yesterday? _____________________
What am I learning and experiencing?

What are my main concerns and predictions for the day?

Were yesterday's concerns/predictions accurate?

How can I apply what I am learning?

Check in 2 (6pm or later)
Have I succeeded in my daily goals so far?

How I feel so far (Emotionally, physically, relationally, etc):

Problems I have encountered and how I am dealing with them:

What was the most difficult part (or time) of the day?

What can I learn to do differently tomorrow (and in the future) to help me stay on track?

CALEB'S JOURNAL, DAY 24 -

We often avoid difficult things – not because we can't do them, but because we've simply gotten used to not trying. As you utilize your willpower and strive for better, you will begin to see how powerful you really are.

Check in 1:

This morning, I tried something new. I made an extra smoothie just for breakfast, which consisted of green beans, kale, a kiwi, green superfood powder mix, and broccoli. Obviously, this was not designed with taste in mind.

I chugged it down fast before my tastebuds knew what was happening. It tasted terrible, but it was terribly good for me. I swigged some cranberry juice afterwards as a chaser, then headed out the door to start my day.

Check in 2:

Believe it or not, I've felt pretty energized by that nasty green vegetable smoothie I made this morning. Maybe I'll try that again. Because, it seems like you're able to pack a lot of punch into a small smoothie once you're willing to compromise taste. My energy levels this afternoon seem to prove it!

I don't think I mentioned my weight this morning, so I'll mention it now. I weighed in at 189.8 lbs. I'm still stuck on the slow downhill road of barely visible results. Today, I will try to do more exercise. I have already done two sets of squats and one set of pushups. I can't slack if I want to reach my weight-loss target, which is 30 pounds! I only have 6 days to go!

JOURNAL, DAY 25

Check in 1 (10am or later)
How many hours of sleep did I get last night? _______________
Did I drink enough water yesterday? __________________________
What am I learning and experiencing?

What are my main concerns and predictions for the day?

Were yesterday's concerns/predictions accurate?

How can I apply what I am learning?

Check in 2 (6pm or later)
Have I succeeded in my daily goals so far?

How I feel so far (Emotionally, physically, relationally, etc):

Problems I have encountered and how I am dealing with them:

What was the most difficult part (or time) of the day?

What can I learn to do differently tomorrow (and in the future) to help me stay on track?

CALEB'S JOURNAL, DAY 25 -

DAILY INSPIRATION:

It is said that "An apple a day keeps the doctor away." While this may not be a literal guarantee, there is some truth to consider in it. When you blend up fresh produce, you are getting vitamins and nutrients in their purest forms. No doubt, this has some effect at keeping us healthy, which in turn, will help us prevent illnesses we might otherwise suffer.

Check in 1:

Today I weighed in at 187.6 pounds. This is excellent! I love to see signs that I'm headed in the right direction!

I slept pretty well too (about 7 hours), and I managed to drink a lot of water throughout the day yesterday. It think it's all part of why I'm feeling more energized today.

Later on, I plan on taking my daughter for a walk around the lake. I may go around twice, which would be over four miles!

Check in 2:

I'm about to take my daughters for a walk. I am finishing up the last of my smoothies. All in all, today has been an extremely easy day for me in almost every way. You've got to love those days.

While on the subject, I should mention that I spoke to a friend today who is trying to take a break from alcohol and caffeine. He told me he is on day 5 of his journey and that he feels more depressed than he has ever felt in his life.

I told him that I felt the same way during my first few days. It's hard to even realize it now, but I got to experience many of those same strong effects when I first began withdrawing from my comforts.

I feel energetic, inspired, and as though my emotions are under control. You cannot put a price tag on this feeling. Also, I'm looking better. When you add up all the bonuses, it's easy to see that healthy living pays off!

JOURNAL, DAY 26

Check in 1 (10am or later)
How many hours of sleep did I get last night? _______________
Did I drink enough water yesterday? _____________________
What am I learning and experiencing?

What are my main concerns and predictions for the day?

Were yesterday's concerns/predictions accurate?

How can I apply what I am learning?

Check in 2 (6pm or later)
Have I succeeded in my daily goals so far?

How I feel so far (Emotionally, physically, relationally, etc):

Problems I have encountered and how I am dealing with them:

What was the most difficult part (or time) of the day?

What can I learn to do differently tomorrow (and in the future) to help me stay on track?

CALEB'S JOURNAL, DAY 26 -

Making healthy decisions doesn't just make us healthy physically, but also, emotionally. It breaks us out of our victim mentalities. Life is more than a matter of what happens to us. It is also a matter of what happens because of us.

Check in 1:

After getting about six and a half hours of sleep last night, I woke and went downstairs to step on the scale. I weighed in at 186.8 pounds! That's exciting!

I prepared my smoothies last night, so now, I just have to grab my thermoses and head out the door. I think that this smoothie fast is also making me better at preparation. Add that to the list of bonuses.

Check in 2:

I'm not sure when, but at some point in my life, I developed an inflammatory response to certain foods. But, over the past 26 days, I have noticed that my stomach feels better than it has felt in years. It's not achy, swollen, or inflamed by whatever bothers it.

I suppose it's just one benefit that only comes over time. And, proof that you cannot base your determination upon immediate results. Most of the great benefits I've seen have been during these past few days – over three long weeks into the plan!

JOURNAL, DAY 27

Check in 1 (10am or later)
How many hours of sleep did I get last night? _______________
Did I drink enough water yesterday? _____________________
What am I learning and experiencing?

What are my main concerns and predictions for the day?

Were yesterday's concerns/predictions accurate?

How can I apply what I am learning?

Check in 2 (6pm or later)
Have I succeeded in my daily goals so far?

How I feel so far (Emotionally, physically, relationally, etc):

Problems I have encountered and how I am dealing with them:

What was the most difficult part (or time) of the day?

What can I learn to do differently tomorrow (and in the future) to help me stay on track?

CALEB'S JOURNAL, DAY 27 -

DAILY INSPIRATION:

It has been said that "A goal is a dream with a deadline." Be glad that you are doing more here than just daydreaming about a better life. You have quantified your objectives and you've made great efforts each day to see that they get done. That's something that's worthy of acknowledgement.

Check in 1:

Last night, I got about 7 hours of sleep. I weighed in this morning at 186.8 lbs. Right now, I am feeling pretty good and satisfied over how easy it's been lately to stick to this plan.

With only three days left to go, I will do my best to keep journaling, although I feel like there haven't been very many noteworthy changes as of late.

Check in 2:

Tomorrow, we are invited over to my parents house for tacos and to celebrate Mother's Day. Right now, I can't tell you how much I wish this plan finished up today. Because, tacos are my weakness. Especially mom and dad's homemade kind!

Tempting though it will be, I have the resolve not to eat food. I've made it this far. Nothing can stop me now! One thing I know is that I'll have the rest of my life to regret certain things, but I'll never regret being strong. This journey has made me realize that. While part of me will be glad when it's over, another part of me will feel sad to see it end.

JOURNAL, DAY 28

Check in 1 (10am or later)
How many hours of sleep did I get last night? _______________
Did I drink enough water yesterday? _________________________
What am I learning and experiencing?

What are my main concerns and predictions for the day?

Were yesterday's concerns/predictions accurate?

How can I apply what I am learning?

Check in 2 (6pm or later)
Have I succeeded in my daily goals so far?

How I feel so far (Emotionally, physically, relationally, etc):

Problems I have encountered and how I am dealing with them:

What was the most difficult part (or time) of the day?

What can I learn to do differently tomorrow (and in the future) to help me stay on track?

CALEB'S JOURNAL, DAY 28 -

Muhammad Ali once said, "Don't count the days, make the days count." Remember that on this journey. Your goal is not simply to pass the time, but to make your time purposeful and beneficial.

Check in 1:

Today, when I stepped on the scale, it felt as though my scale was permanently stuck at 186.8. Really… it's kind of hard to fathom how it's possible not to lose even an ounce in 72 hours, especially when I'm not putting any solid foods into my body!

This morning, I felt some small traces of arthritis pain. It leads me to believe that there still must be something in my smoothies that my body doesn't agree with. In these last few days, I'll have to pay close attention to whatever might be causing it.

For the time being, I have done some stomach exercises and squats. I will do more as the day goes on. Right now, we're on our way to my parents' house to celebrate Mother's day. The real trials will begin soon!

Check in 2:

Just as I predicted, it was an extremely rough day. There were so many amazing types of food on the buffet table that I began to wonder if I should end my fast early. But, I didn't do it. I stayed strong!

And as usual, when it was all over and when we were putting leftover food back into the refrigerator, I did not feel a sense of regret for choosing to stay strong. I felt proud of myself for being able to resist even the strongest of temptations.

I can't tell you why I've felt tired and lethargic all day. It's obviously not from anything I've eaten. All I can say is that I'm glad I got to take a nap at my parents' house. It felt so much better after crashing out on their couch for an hour!

JOURNAL, DAY 29

Check in 1 (10am or later)
How many hours of sleep did I get last night? _______________
Did I drink enough water yesterday? _________________________
What am I learning and experiencing?

What are my main concerns and predictions for the day?

Were yesterday's concerns/predictions accurate?

How can I apply what I am learning?

Check in 2 (6pm or later)
Have I succeeded in my daily goals so far?

How I feel so far (Emotionally, physically, relationally, etc):

Problems I have encountered and how I am dealing with them:

What was the most difficult part (or time) of the day?

What can I learn to do differently tomorrow (and in the future) to help me stay on track?

CALEB'S JOURNAL, DAY 29 -

Babe Ruth once said, "Yesterday's home runs don't win today's games." On this journey, you'll make great strides. But, no matter how great, your goal doesn't change. You can't earn a break from trying simply because you feel ahead. There is no getting ahead. There is only what's in front of you now.

Check in 1:

This morning, I was pleased to see that I weighed 185.5 pounds! Awesome. Things continue to head in the right direction! With my smoothies from yesterday already made, I head off to work feeling much more energized than I did yesterday.

Tomorrow will be my last day! I can't believe it. Nor can I help but think about how far I've come and how glad I am to have stayed the course. It makes me feel confident – not only that I can set a big goal and keep it, but that it is within my power to stay feeling good and healthy in the future.

Check in 2:

This evening has been tough, though I've seen tougher. Around 6pm, I had to watch my work partner scarf down a pork burrito from Chipotle. I suppose the day may never come when a smoothie looks more enticing than a giant pork burrito.

A few people at work have told me that I look better and are interested in knowing more about what I've been doing. For me, this is very encouraging. For one, because it's better than when they just think you're crazy. But also, because it is a reminder that this plan is paying off.

Today I realize that my pants are no longer tight on me. I need to use a different hole on my belt. That is a good feeling to. The good news is that, contrary to what I thought earlier, I may not need a new wardrobe after all!

JOURNAL, DAY 30

Check in 1 (10am or later)
How many hours of sleep did I get last night? _______________
Did I drink enough water yesterday? ____________________
What am I learning and experiencing?

What are my main concerns and predictions for the day?

Were yesterday's concerns/predictions accurate?

How can I apply what I am learning?

Check in 2 (6pm or later)
Have I succeeded in my daily goals so far?

How I feel so far (Emotionally, physically, relationally, etc):

Problems I have encountered and how I am dealing with them:

What was the most difficult part (or time) of the day?

What can I learn to do differently tomorrow (and in the future) to help me stay on track?

CALEB'S JOURNAL, DAY 30 -

DAILY INSPIRATION:

It has been said that "If you obey all the rules, you'll miss all the fun." While this humorous statement could be taken many ways, we take it to mean that there is a lot to gain by being different. Look at what's considered normal. Eating junk. Sitting around. Feeling lethargic. Question: do you really want to be normal? While you may be going against the flow, or, "breaking the rules" of society, you'll be "experiencing the fun" that comes from being a healthy type of different. Don't let people make you feel weird because you're stepping outside the box.

Check in 1:

This is my very last day, and I'm so excited! Soon, I'll be able to say that I did what I set out to do. Yeah, it's been a wild ride. And, while it's still not over yet, the end is right at my fingertips.

This morning, I weighed 186 pounds even. I got about 6 hours of sleep due to kids crying in the middle of the night. I have another softball game to go to later, so I'll be getting my light exercise then. I also plan on drinking lots of water throughout the day.

Check in 2: <u>VIDEO</u>

I've just run two miles and finished my second smoothie for the day. I'm almost ready to head to bed. Being only a few short hours away from the finish line, I have some bittersweet feelings. It feels good think of not having so many restrictions, and yet, it saddens me to think of the positive changes ending. I don't want that to happen.

So, as I wean myself back onto food, I plan to continue including smoothies as part of my everyday diet. I also plan to eat things that will not be too hard on my system (such as oatmeal, fruit, vegetables, etc).

As I stride towards the finish line, I make a promise to myself. Someday soon, I will do this again. I've seen how how beneficial it has been. I've seen that my normal life needs to be broken up by periods of restoration.

Good night, world. Tomorrow, I wake a new man – transformed by this incredible journey.

MY WEIGHT CHART -

DAY	Weight	Hardest Part of day
1	208	11am-9pm
2	204	6pm
3	199.8	2pm - 6pm
4	198.6	6pm-midnight
5	197.8	2pm
6	196	2pm
7	195.3	N/A
8	199.8	N/A
9	199	7pm
10	195	N/A
11	196.4	N/A
12	191.6	N/A
13	191.4	2pm
14	191.4	6pm
15	191	N/A
16	N/A	N/A
17	N/A	N/A
18	189.4	2pm
19	N/A	N/A
20	189.2	N/A
21	189.6	N/A
22	189.2	N/A
23	191.2	8pm
24	189.8	4pm

25	187.6	N/A
26	186.8	6pm
27	186.8	N/A
28	186.6	3pm
29	185.5	N/A
30	186	N/A